the
ROCKSTAR
Remedy

the ROCKSTAR *Remedy*

A ROCK & ROLL DOCTOR'S PRESCRIPTION
FOR LIVING A LONG, HEALTHY LIFE

DR. GABRIELLE FRANCIS
WITH STACY BAKER MASAND

WITH ARTIST INTERVIEWS BY JULIE PANEBIANCO,
LONN M. FRIEND, AND STACY BAKER MASAND

<tt>HARPER WAVE</tt>

This book is written as a source of information only. The information contained in this book should by no means be considered a substitute for the advice of a qualified medical professional, who should always be consulted before beginning any new diet, exercise, or other health program.

All efforts have been made to ensure the accuracy of the information contained in this book as of the date published. The author and the publisher expressly disclaim responsibility for any adverse effects arising from the use or application of the information contained herein.

FIRST EDITION

Photography by Mick Rock and Danny Clinch, unless otherwise indicated.

Record sleeve image throughout by donatas1205/Shutterstock, Inc.

Designed by William Ruoto

Library of Congress Cataloging-in-Publication Data

Francis, Gabrielle.

The rockstar remedy : a rock & roll doctor's prescription for living a long, healthy life / Dr. Gabrielle Francis.

pages   cm

ISBN 978-0-06-231060-6

1. Health. 2. Nutrition. 3. Naturopathy. 4. Detoxification (Health) 5. Celebrities—Health and hygiene. 6. Rock musicians—Health and hygiene. I. Title.

RA776.F83   2014

613.2—dc23   2014028188

14 15 16 17 18   OV/RRD   10 9 8 7 6 5 4 3 2 1

This book is dedicated to the "rock star" in you!

That rebellious spirit that refuses to settle for the status quo . . .

The fire within that ignites transformation in body, mind, and spirit . . .

The desire to create the life of your dreams . . .

So that you can fulfill your true destiny . . .

Join me on the adventure . . .

CONTENTS

PART THREE: Nourish and Revive

PART FOUR: Heal, Restore, and Recover

THE OPENING ACT

The terms "healthy living" and "rock star" are rarely used in the same sentence. In fact when most of us think of the rock & roll lifestyle, the first word that comes to mind is "excess"—too much partying, too many wild nights, too much sex, drugs, and rock & roll.

The truth is that while all of those things do indeed exist, those of us who have managed to sustain careers in music that span many decades have at some point found a way of eating, exercising, relaxing, and sleeping that keeps our bodies functioning at their peak and our minds at their creative best.

You may be surprised to learn that the rock & roll lifestyle is not that much different than that of a very intense business traveler: living out of airports, taxis, and hotels; dashing from appointment to appointment; working very late; getting up too early; answering emails; taking phone calls; and eating on the run. Sound familiar? Apart from the two hours onstage performing, the stresses of life on the road may be very similar to those you find in your own life.

I don't want it to sound as though being a musician is more

stressful than other jobs, but rarely being in the same place for more than one night in a row does make eating well, exercising, and sleeping a challenge that takes thought, planning, and a bit of tenacity.

When I met Dr. Gabrielle Francis, I was twenty-five pounds heavier, borderline diabetic, fatigued all day, and had permanent acid reflux. I had trouble sleeping, caught every cold and flu that came near me, and generally felt pretty crappy most of the time.

Dr. Francis showed me that by altering what I ate, exercising regularly, and supplementing with some nutrients that my body was lacking, I could shed pounds, get my blood sugar under control, sleep better, boost my immune system, and generally feel more energetic. She taught me that living a rock & roll life didn't have to mean being unhealthy. The recommendations she shares in this book have helped me feel stronger onstage and more present, focused, and creative in my professional and personal

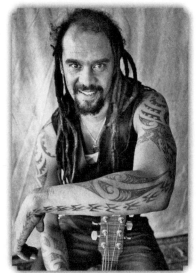

MICHAEL FRANTI
(DANNY CLINCH)

life. All of this has led to my feeling happier, healthier, more youthful, and more inspired than I ever would have imagined after twenty-five years of life on tour.

In this book, Dr. Francis will show you how to make the same kinds of simple and effective changes that will enable you to feel your best and most vibrant so that you can step confidently onto the most important stage of all . . . *your life.*

—Michael Franti, of Michael Franti & Spearhead

SOUND CHECK: YOU ARE A ROCK STAR

I am not your average physician. I do not have a traditional medical office or wear a crisp white lab coat or write prescriptions on an Rx pad. My remedies come from Mother Nature, not pharmaceuticals. And for the past thirty years, I have been practicing natural medicine, chiropractic, acupuncture, and massage while traveling from city to city around the country and around the globe. My clients have some of the most demanding jobs in the world: They're rock stars.

"I surround myself with people who make health a priority. When you are healthy, your music becomes healthy with it. When your spirit is strong and you support the body and mind, the art follows. That has been a key factor in how I live my life on the road and how everyone I surround myself with lives, too. The priority is being healthy."

—SAUL SIMON-MacWILLIAMS, KEYBOARDIST, INGRID MICHAELSON

I work backstage, in hotel rooms, at music festivals, and on planes and buses. I am a rock & roll doctor. That means that the plan I've created for you in this book has been road-tested on some of the most extreme lifestyles in the world.

While there's a lot of fantasy surrounding the way my clients live, the truth is that myths are much sexier than the facts. The best-kept secret of the music industry is probably the one that will shock you the most—the majority of the musicians I know are as full-on committed to their health as they are to partying, like, well, *rock stars*.

"I play rock & roll, I play punk, and I play hip-hop. You want to stay in shape so that you can communicate that basically your body is your instrument. And the same way that I will polish my guitar and take care of that . . . you sort of have to treat your body that same way."

—KIRK DOUGLAS, GUITARIST, **THE ROOTS**

Most of the time, that is. As is the case with your life, there are always outside influences in musicians' lives that set them back a bit, making it impossible to be perfect in their goals for healthy living. After all, rock stars lead highly stressful lives, especially when they are on tour. The glamour you see onstage is far from their experience on the road. Their hard-core schedules require long days that end at 4 a.m. and the days, which can include an 8 a.m. lobby call, are filled with travel between cities, little sleep or exercise, back-to-back media interviews, and preparation for the next show. Now, imagine keeping that intense pace over twenty-four months: U2's 360 tour launched in 2009, consisted of several hundred concerts, and spanned more than two dozen countries and six continents over two years. (Cher, yes, Cher, in her sixties, has also kept up one of the longest tour schedules ever, performing to over 5.88 million fans in twenty countries in 2004–2005.) A touring rock star's daily life is extremely stressful on the body and mind. They must have the stamina and endurance of a professional athlete to keep up with the grueling pace. Maintaining their health is the only way to achieve that. Even if all they can manage on the road is stress management and minimizing the harm they are doing to their bodies, when it comes to health, even a little effort is better than nothing! Eventually, when the tour ends and the pendulum swings back from the extreme to the "normal" range, they are able to focus on repairing and rebuilding their bodies.

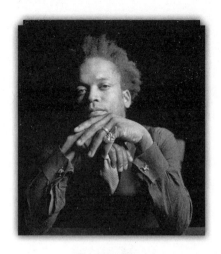

KIRK DOUGLAS
(DANNY CLINCH)

YOU FACE THE SAME CHALLENGES AS ROCK STARS

"I got back together with one of my old bands, Los Desaparecidos. We're all in our early thirties now. And the last time we did it, we were, like, twenty-one. So after, we'd get up in the morning, no one can walk, no one can bend over. Everyone's necks are all crooked. It is a super-intense workout. We've known people who have gotten even more energetic as they have gotten older, like Bruce. How the hell is he doing this? He's sixty-whatever years old, sliding on his knees across the stage and doing a three-hour show and killing it. That's rock & roll, baby! That's the real deal."

—CONOR OBERST, SINGER, SONGWRITER, BRIGHT EYES,
LOS DESAPARECIDOS

My guess is that your life can get pretty crazy, too, and probably also follows a similar ebb-and-flow of extremes. Whether you're a working professional or a full-time parent, you are in demand. The pressures you face may vary in intensity by the minutes or hours or days, and last weeks,

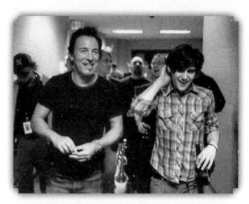

**BRUCE SPRINGSTEEN AND CONOR OBERST
(DANNY CLINCH)**

months, and even years. And like life, your health exists on this type of spectrum, with complete vitality, energy, and happiness on one end and sickness and disease on the other. Most of us, celebrities included, are somewhere in the middle, moving toward "perfect health" when we take good care of ourselves, and toward sickness when we don't. My goal for you, the same one I hold for my rock star clients, is to constantly shift away from the disease side of the spectrum and toward good health. In other words, *my focus is to keep you balanced.* Look at stars like Carlos Santana, Mick Jagger, Madonna, Bruce Springsteen, and Tina Turner. They are living proof that a balanced approach can keep you vibrant and energetic decade after decade.

Balancing the *enjoyment* of life's pleasures with being mindful of your *health* is the secret to achieving vitality when you're living a demanding, work-hard, play-hard life. And it's also the key to achieving your health goals.

If you are like me, my clients, or 95 percent of the people who try mainstream diets and fail, you are not perfect. The traditional one-size-fits-all plans don't work because we are not all one size. Each of us thinks, acts, and lives differently—we may be able to conform to a one-size-fits-all approach for a short time, but over the long erm, we will revert back to who we are as individuals and "fail" in the one-size-fits-all program.

"Music since the beginning has always been our vehicle to speak to the higher power. Cavemen howling to the skies, slaves working in the cotton fields singing the gospel hymns, cultures of Latin origins like mine . . . everywhere the same message. Singing to God to get through the day. The gospel became R&B and the blues became rock & roll. Once you separate spirit from the music, you're dead."
—RUDY SARZO, BASSIST, OZZY OSBOURNE, QUIET RIOT, WHITESNAKE

You are unique, and so is your situation, by the hour and the day, the week, and the month. Different people have different rhythms. That's normal. And that is exactly the reason *The Rockstar Remedy* approach is so successful: *It's all about you.* It meets you where you are, based on your life situation, from your current state of health to your career, your relationships, and your goals. My plan teaches you to realistically assess the essence of who you are, where you are now, and what your needs will be in the future. It then gives you the tools to make the appropriate changes for your lifestyle.

Looking at health from this balanced perspective gives you a real shot at the vitality, focus, and level of performance that a full-on rock star life demands. This is the philosophy I use with my clients. It's how I live as a practicing natural medicine physician. And it's what I'm about to teach you.

MY STORY FROM NATURAL MEDICINE DOCTOR TO "TOUR DOCTOR"

My first gig treating rock stars came when I was fresh out of massage school, a ripe nineteen years old. Around that time, a cousin who worked in concert production called me and said that the hugest name in rock & roll wanted a massage in Cleveland and she had volunteered me. Sure, I was in a state of shock, but I gladly accepted the offer. Weirdly enough, I was not nervous. I arrived at the Coliseum with my massage table and confidence in check, secretly looking forward to the massive parties backstage.

To my dismay, backstage was surprisingly quite quiet. All the artists were in their private dressing rooms and keeping to themselves. Instead of sex, drugs, and, of course, rock & roll, there was meditation music and a spread of organic, vegetarian food, which in those days was very rare and almost unheard-of. There was not an ounce of alcohol backstage. The most intoxicating beverage was Coca-Cola. I was blown away. You mean no one was going to be tearing up hotel rooms? Where were the groupies? Instead, I met their wives. The myth was shattered!

One of the artists, the sax player, had transformed his dressing room into an Indian temple, complete with incense and candles—he had replaced the placard with his stage name on the door with the "spiritual" name his guru gave him. I knocked on the door and was welcomed in to where he sat inside, meditating beneath a picture of his Indian guru, who stared at me throughout the massage. As the day went on, I met the rest of the band. Each artist was so thoughtful and down-to-earth. I was taken by their humility and realness. This was not what I had expected. It was so relaxed and focused, a true ego-free zone.

Most of the band got massages from me, and a medical doctor gave each member B_{12} shots to help with extra energy for the big performance. And it was big. The band put on a super four-hour marathon show that night as I watched from backstage in awe. The group gave energy to the audience, and I saw how the audience fed appreciation and more energy back to them. In turn, the band got high on the energy from the crowd. It seemed like it could go on forever. And it almost did. The band only left the stage because the venue told them they had to go.

I will never forget that night as I saw the power of music elevate the energy of a theater to a higher vibration. It's no wonder that some people feel that going to a concert can be like a religious experience. In that moment, I decided it would be one of my religions, too. It would blend very well with my Catholic upbringing. I was taught to revere saints, so why not add a few more? There was Jimi Hendrix, Patron Saint of the Wah-Wah Pedal; Santana, the Archangel of Long Instrumental Grooves; Keith Richards, Holy Father of the Rhythm Guitar; and, of course, Our Lady Madonna.

After the show, the band asked me to tour with them as their massage therapist. I had to say no because I was committed to finishing medical school, a decision I regretted for a very long time. Luckily, I had the chance again almost seventeen years later. In the meantime, my decision to massage the band that night changed the course of my life. Production companies stayed in contact with me and booked me whenever bands toured through my cities for the next seventeen years.

THE RUDE AWAKENING

I remember sitting in naturopathic school with other students and hearing them talk about how their future practices would be.

They would say things like "If my patients eat at McDonald's, I won't work with them," or "I can only work with people who are open to raw food and vegetarianism," or "Coffee is the root of all things evil and my patients will not drink it."

It led me to wonder how these future doctors were going to pay off their student loan bills. Who would be their patients? It hadn't crossed my mind that my first practice would be touring with rock bands and I would have this dilemma, too.

When I graduated from seventeen years of medical school, I was so burned out that I decided to take a few months' sabbatical and do the traveling I had always wanted to do. So I sold my possessions, closed my chiropractic practice, and headed to Europe with a backpack and no hotel reservation. Several months later, one of the bands I had worked with previously got wind I was in Europe. They wanted someone to go on tour and do some natural medicine for them. What a day it was to take a taxi from the youth hostel in Paris where I was sharing a room with six people to the very swanky Paris hotel where I would meet the group!

I had my massage tables sent to Europe along with a natural medicine pharmacy of herbs, vitamins, and acupuncture needles. I was excited about the prospect of incorporating all of the healing modalities I had learned into one practice.

I was in for a rude awakening! My visions of the ultimate natural medicine practice quickly vanished. After Paris, the band headed to Amsterdam. Need I say more? It became clear that these musicians were just as committed to revelry and debauchery as they were to their health. The preventive medicine I knew turned into harm reduction for hangovers and sexually transmitted disease. What to do? Although this wasn't the kind of natural medicine I intended to practice, I put my judgments aside and learned to use my medicines any chance I got. As a doctor, I needed to experience this. This is how I learned to meet people where they are and make small changes where I could. I discovered it is possible to be healthy and have a lot of fun, too.

Eventually I returned to the United States and began practicing holistic medicine in a proper practice in San Francisco and now in New York City. Through these practices and my interactions with my clients, I began to realize that the issues of "normal" people were very much the same as the issues and circumstances faced by my celebrity clients. As I treated more and more patients with crazy work schedules, demanding parental duties, and an array of social obligations, I realized that just about everyone is living extreme lifestyles these days. That's why it's so important to take advantage of opportunities to improve our health wherever they appear. I found myself using the same "harm reduction" techniques and negotiations with my patients as I had used on tour to keep musicians functioning when they were under the stress of grueling schedules. I learned to teach patients that they could improve the quality of their lives without changing the essence of who they are and what they love to do. This is the philosophy of *The Rockstar Remedy*: improve the quality of your life and health so that you can keep doing what you love to do.

WHY ROCK STARS MAKE INCREDIBLE SELF-HELP GURUS

Aside from the fact that musicians face many of the same stressors as we do, why should we look to them as models of health and wellness? Let me give you two reasons.

1 Rock stars don't believe in aging. People always talk about how great musicians look for their age.

Think about it—Madonna, Mick Jagger, Bruce Springsteen—none of them seems to look their age, and all of them can perform with as much energy and intensity as they did decades ago. You know why? Because rock stars don't buy into the idea of aging. Legendary artists don't wake up every morning thinking about the birth date listed on their driver's license. They couldn't care less. To be honest with you, neither could I.

Most people define their health based on what statistics tell them should be happening to their bodies at a certain age. But just because you are older doesn't mean a certain condition is normal for you. Is arthritis common for someone who is seventy years old? Yes. But it's not normal. I want you to consider where you want to be in terms of your health, regardless of your age or current medical situation, and I will help you achieve that state. The program in this book will stretch your imagination about what's possible for your optimal health, raise your expectations about how incredible you can look and feel, and enhance your longevity in the same way rock icons have learned to live forever.

"I am inspired daily by the younger generation, both creatively and personally. Most of my friends are half my age. Those are the people who have bold new ideas."
—DAVE NAVARRO, GUITARIST, JANE'S ADDICTION

"You have to get serious with life at some point. With most people, it doesn't happen until they're old. When you're a teenager, you just deny it. Forty years of denial and when this teen finally hits fifty, he's confronted with a doctor who tells him the truth."

—STEVEN TYLER, SINGER, SONGWRITER,
MULTI-INSTRUMENTALIST, AEROSMITH

2 Rock stars are revolutionaries. They realize that the negative experiences in life can be even more powerful and transformative than the positive ones. And people with revolutionary spirits are generally willing to take responsibility for the negative places they have reached in their lives and make positive efforts toward change.

That's why so many rock stars are drawn to natural medicine. They don't think inside the box, and through years of trial and error, they've learned that they can't make their symptoms go away with chemical treatments or a handful of pills. Most of the artists in this book have experienced some sort of physical issue that has led them to alternative medicine. Once there, they realized it works. The program in this book will challenge you to turn your health obstacles into opportunities for healing in all areas of your life and give you personal tools for creating lasting changes.

My job is to ignite the possibility of change within you, but how you approach this journey is as unique as you are. You may read this book from start to finish and gather new ideas; you might use it as a reference when you need to address a specific symptom or detox from a busy time; or you might want to flip through the "Bonus Tracks" at the end of each chapter— which are filled with anecdotes from rock stars like you—to get inspired to make healthy changes. No matter how you use it, as of this moment you no longer have to choose between being healthy and enjoying your life. If you dream of feeling recharged, rejuvenated, and reinspired; if you long for happiness, confidence, and peace of mind; know that it can happen, regardless of your age or circumstances. If you are ready to live your life to the fullest, look no further.

PART ONE

THE RxSTAR REMEDY PHILOSOPHY

CHAPTER 1

YOU DON'T HAVE TO MISS THE PARTY: THE 90/10 RULE

W ho says you can't have your cake and eat it, too? Certainly not me.

> "Life is to be enjoyed and to have fun. We have these ideas that being healthy is hard and not fun, but I don't think so. People have this idea eating healthy is not fun, but once you retrain yourself and start to eat good food, you start to realize that that's the good food. This other stuff is just crap. You start to realize that you can have a wonderful, fun life and you can be healthy."
> —JESSY GREENE, VIOLINIST, PINK, THE FOO FIGHTERS

I'm all about indulgence in balance. Do the things that bring you joy while being mindful of your health. That's balance. When you do what you love, you're more likely to succeed in the long run. When you anchor your health decisions around your preferences and your lifestyle, you're happier and healthier.

I'm the last person to ask you to overhaul your lifestyle, change who you are, or never have fun again. That's a recipe for failure, plus who wants to live that way? The key to making sustainable changes is to start small and build a strong foundation. You will begin by giving yourself a clean slate to start from (that's the RxStar Detox) and then build nourishing habits and make smarter choices. We will cover how to select the best nutrient-dense foods for your needs, exercise optimally, and reduce the health hazards of some of your less-than-perfect choices. The entire plan is designed for and built around you.

Throughout the book, I'll also offer you my damage mitigation strategies, called "Harm Reduction Techniques," which are my signature methods for making your bad habits a little less destructive. For example, I had a client who refused to give up coffee on his detox, so we made a deal: he could drink one cup of coffee per day as long as he added certain spices that reduce its acidity. He got his caffeine and I got him to stick to his detox plan without quitting. These Harm Reduction tricks work because they fit into your lifestyle and make the program achievable. They keep your goals in check by offsetting the negative impact of unhealthy choices, like a late-night ice-cream binge or a morning bagel run. In this program, you aren't expected to be perfect. You're expected to be the healthiest version of you.

MEET THE 90/10 RULE

It so simple, it can be your plan for life: 10 percent of the time you do what you want. You don't worry or limit yourself about the food or indulgences at events, concerts, parties, restaurants, or ice-cream runs with your kids. You can participate in, and on occasion relish in, the extravagances of life. This means enjoying a hard-earned happy hour cocktail during the week or a lazy Saturday spent in your pajamas or an occasional all-night party with friends—as long as you're making healthy choices the other 90 percent of the time. This is what I call "maintenance mode," and it begins after you've detoxed and begun to practice new healthy habits on a daily basis.

> "It is really more about not denying yourself the pleasures of life. But don't be an idiot. Because you can't have both the pleasures of life and be a complete idiot about it without ending up in a place where you are not going to like the way you look or feel. Nothing is built that way. If you are going to be excessive in a way that is going to be detrimental, you have to find a balance."
>
> **—RUSSELL SIMINS, DRUMMER,**
> ## JON SPENCER BLUES EXPLOSION

When you follow this simple guideline on a daily, weekly, monthly, or even yearly basis—90 percent of the time—you'll discover that you feel so incredible living a healthy lifestyle that the 10 percent of the time when you *do* let your hair down, you'll be keenly aware of the toll it takes on your body. My patients always report back to me that during the 10 percent of the time when they're indulging, they notice a big difference in their bodies. Whether they splurged on a decadent meal, too many drinks, or simply neglected to sleep or exercise properly for a while—they look and feel terrible. These consequences of making less healthy choices are physical proof of how much benefit your body gets from your efforts the other 90 percent of the time. After all, who wants to feel less than great any more than 10 percent of the time? Experiencing the difference in how your body feels when you don't take care of yourself versus when you do serves as its own motivation for sticking to the plan.

Staying consistent with your diet and fitness plans pays off not only when you're "being healthy"—it also allows you more freedom and less guilt during the 10 percent of the time you let loose. For example, many of my celebrity clients try to live within healthy food, fitness, and lifestyle guidelines while on tour and at home, and save their 10 percent "relapse time" for parties, events, dinners, or vacation. Maintaining a strict adherence to the rules while they're intensely focused on their work allows them to truly enjoy themselves and be sociable when they want to be. This is one of the main reasons my clients stick to my program. Your odds of success are far greater because you don't sacrifice or sabotage your lifestyle to keep your mind, body, and spirit in check.

THE 90/10 RULE? WHAT ABOUT 70/30?

"My favorite philosophy that I made up is an analogy to banking and your body and your mind as you get older. If you don't make deposits you can't make withdrawals, and that is it. If you are just going to glide through life eating pizzas and hamburgers and drinking, when you go to make a withdrawal, you are not going to have a lot of money in the bank."

—RICHARD MANITOBA, AKA "HANDSOME DICK," PUNK ROCK SINGER, THE DICTATORS

THE ROCKSTAR REMEDY

Hey, no one is keeping score but you. Maybe you are on the 80/20 or the 70/30 plan. This is your life and your regimen. Your challenge will be to become your own health advocate. So when you notice that 30 percent of the time you don't feel so great, your energy is low, and symptoms like headaches, fatigue, or insomnia return, check in with yourself. How much are you sleeping? What are you eating? Are you getting enough exercise or activity? How stressed-out are you?

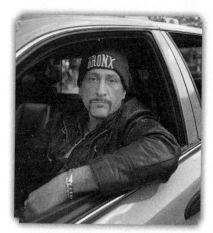

HANDSOME DICK MANITOBA
(DANNY CLINCH)

You may be someone who's willing to sacrifice feeling great every day to the rigorous demands of your work schedule or child care, or because you simply have a hard time saying "no" to every social invitation. But when you consistently make your health your last priority, your body accumulates toxins. So if your idea of balance falls more in the 70-30 or 60-40 range, you may need to do my detox plan more frequently to restore balance because your life doesn't fall mostly in the maintenance mode. Remember that spectrum of health we talked about? Keep in mind that in order to stay on the healthy side of the spectrum, the number of positive choices you make must outweigh the negative ones.

"I do total silence for ten minutes right after a show. . . . As my ears ring out and all my energies start to come back to earth, I find peace in that ten minutes, then it's time to party!"
—TOMMY LEE, DRUMMER, MÖTLEY CRÜE

Remember, even small changes in your lifestyle move you away from the disease end of the spectrum and propel you toward the healthy end. This is why a balanced approach to health works long-term. And when you slip up or need to cheat the system, your arsenal of Harm Reduction Techniques will keep you from losing too much footing. When it comes to balance, we're not striving for 50-50; doing anything halfway doesn't get you anywhere. True balance is about making your health a priority while pursuing what brings you joy in life. When you allow this mindset to guide the choices you make, you'll find that you don't have to choose between abundant health, a productive life, and the ability to enjoy that life with the people you love.

CHAPTER 2

THE RxSTAR REMEDY REVOLUTION

Rock stars on tour have to be on top of their game. Their demanding lifestyles don't give them the luxury of abusing their bodies the way the rest of society does. To perform at such intense levels, night after night, for months on end, artists must become as vigilant about their health as professional athletes. But unlike the pros, rock stars don't have an injured reserve list. And the economics of the tours don't leave much room for play. With shows lasting two to three hours and backstage entertaining going into the next morning, rock stars who get wrecked each night threaten to mess up the timing of their entire schedule. If bands can't play, they get pulled off the road and don't get paid. This puts extreme pressure on them to take care of themselves. When was the last time *your* schedule was that hectic?

"To me, a rock star is somebody like Bono, Sting, and Springsteen—once you fulfill your passion or dreams, you kick into the next level, and that's fulfilling your destiny. What's the destiny of man? To take care of each other, like Bono said in 'One.' Carry each other. Destiny is not choosing a profession. Success is a gift, and those who get it are inspired and required to give back."

—RUDY SARZO, BASSIST, OZZY OSBOURNE, QUIET RIOT, WHITESNAKE

The irony is that musicians are often perceived as killing themselves with their crazy lifestyles. But the truth is that we *non*–rock stars are the ones fueling our bodies with toxic chemicals and hard living. I call this "soda pop" culture. Many of my non-celebrity clients push themselves just as hard as the artists I work with, but don't take nearly as good care of themselves. When they see me for the first time, many of them are exhausted, sleep-deprived, stressed out, and depressed. Their diets consist mainly of processed, packaged, or fast food; tons of sugary drinks; lots of caffeine; and whatever else they can grab on the run that doesn't take too much time away from other commitments. Their relationships are suffering. Emotionally, they feel out of whack. And their brains and bodies are having a hard time coping with it all.

CHANGING HEALTH PARADIGMS

While the rock star life hasn't always been synonymous with clean living, a lot has changed in the past twenty years. In fact, the industry's journey toward better health mirrors the significant shifts in health and food paradigms that have taken place over the past few decades.

To truly understand how radically our thinking about health has changed in more recent years, let's look back to the 1950s, when processed food products were thought to be so far superior to whole foods that women were encouraged to feed their babies formula rather than breastfeed. Food had become corporatized, and we lost any sense of connection between food, the environment, and our health—it was just about variety on the grocery store shelves and the convenience of packaged and frozen meals. Even in the sixties, women were still smoking and drinking while they were pregnant, which wasn't considered dangerous because doctors were smoking, too. No one had linked cigarettes to lung disease. In fact, diseases were thought to be the result of infection or bad genes, so your lifestyle made little difference.

By the seventies, attitudes toward health began to shift. The organic movement began spreading globally. Government agencies and international committees began to more rigorously research and regulate systems of food and agriculture. At the same time, doctors and scientists were beginning to understand a new model of disease: perhaps we were more than just victims of our genes. Researchers studied the health effects of environmental toxins. They questioned whether specific types of food were related to issues like heart disease and diabetes, and they looked at the negative impact of smoking on our lungs. From this point on, a revolution in health happened in five stages:

1. Recognition of the Body-Mind Connection

A new science called psychoneuroimmunology was created when doctors and researchers decided to find out whether this mind-body connection espoused by the yoga crowd was more than a "new age" idea. They knew that the endocrine, gastrointestinal, immune, and nervous systems all start as the same tissue in utero and later differentiate as we grow and develop.

But what they didn't focus on was how these systems might continue to communicate with one another. During this time in medicine, doctors were still separated by their disciplines, so if you had a nervous system issue, you saw a neurologist, but if you experienced gastrointestinal problems, you went to a GI specialist. There was an immunologist for immune disorders. For every condition there was a specialist, but no one was considering how the body functions as a whole.

Scientists studying psychoneuroimmunology began digging into research on neurotransmitters like serotonin. Previously, serotonin was simply considered a "happy molecule" that floated around in the brain; this research revealed what we know to be true today: it is actually a systemic communicator between all systems in your body. Ninety-five percent of serotonin is produced inside your digestive tract in something called gut-associated lymphatic tissue, or GALT—not your brain. Serotonin thus regulates your hormones, your digestive system, your immune system, and your nervous system. In other words, it's not just a happy molecule. There is a direct connection between the health of our gut and our emotions (hence the term "gut feelings"). In fact, the gut has an entire nervous system of its own. That's why currently, many digestive conditions such as irritable bowel syndrome are treated with antidepressants. Since the 1970s this new scientific field has continued to prove that the mind-body connection is valid and not some "new age" ideology. Our body affects the mind and the mind affects the body; this huge shift in thinking has had major implications for our health.

2. Functional Medicine: Patient-Centered

A new paradigm and system of medicine called Functional Medicine began in the late 1970s and early '80s, founded by the incredible Dr. Jeffrey Bland, who studied nutritional biochemistry. This method addresses the underlying causes of disease using a systems-oriented approach and engages both the patient and practitioner in a therapeutic partnership. By shifting the traditional disease-centered focus of medical practice to a systems-based model, functional medicine addresses the whole person, not just an isolated set of symptoms. Practitioners spend time with their patients, listening to their histories and looking at genetic, environmental, and lifestyle factors that can influence long-term health and chronic disease. In this way, functional medicine supports the unique expression of health and vitality for each individual.

The foundations of functional medicine began with a new approach to treatment of the liver and the gut. The foundational focus centered around improving the ability of the liver to detoxify and the ability of the gut to absorb nutrients. This research has become the basis for much of what we know about gut health and detoxification today.

3. The Human Genome Project

Another major shift in the way we approach health care began in 1990 with the Human Genome Project, funded by the National Institutes of Health. It was originally believed that each of us is born with a genetic blueprint that is permanent—your blueprint probably looked a lot like your parents' blueprint, and there wasn't much hope of changing your genetic future. The conventional wisdom was that you were destined to develop the same diseases that ailed your mother and father.

The Human Genome Project took researchers more than a decade to complete. The goal was to isolate human genes in order to understand how each gene works individually. As new insights were discovered about the ways in which different genes function and can be turned "off" or "on" by environmental factors, scientists began to focus on the dynamic quality of our genetic blueprint. External influences can make all the difference in whether or not you develop the diseases that plagued your parents and grandparents. For example, you can be in an unhealthy physical state, but if you expose your body to high-quality food, empowering thoughts, and healthy emotions, you can create a more positive outcome in your body than if you expose yourself to low-quality foods, sabotaging thoughts, and unhealthy emotions. External influences and information from food, toxins, thoughts, and emotions are now seen as major contributors in determining whether your genes express health or disease.

4. Alternative Medicine Works

The seventies were a time when many ideas about health that had been evolving for hundreds of years began to gel together. Traditional doctors began exploring treatment modalities developed in other areas of the world and subjecting those treatments to the rigors of peer-reviewed medical studies. In some cases the studies indicated that these alternative treatments provided tremendous benefits, and so these "alternative" treatments started to gain some traction in the medical community and with the public.

Acupuncture is one such example. Acupuncture and and other forms of Chinese medicine were first brought to the United States by immigrants, but remained relatively unknown to the general public until the visit of Richard Nixon to China in 1972. At that time a reporter traveling with the president wrote about his experiences with acupuncture and Chinese medicine and its powerful effects. Soon, mainstream America followed in his footsteps.

Around the same time naturopathic medicine became a legitimate, viable alternative medical system. Naturopathic medicine is founded on traditional beliefs in the power of the body to heal itself. Unlike conventional medicine, which is most often focused on treating the symptoms a patient is experiencing, naturopathic medicine is focused on finding and treating the underlying causes of the disease. Treatments combine diet and noninvasive therapies to stimulate the healing process and vitality of the patient.

Chiropractic, an alternative discipline that developed in North America in the 1800s, also began to receive funding for serious study in the 1970s, which allowed the field to become a true science. The foundation of chiropractic philosophy is that the structure of the body affects the function. Working with spinal and structural alignment may improve the function of the nervous system, circulatory system, lymphatic system, and more.

The momentum of these separate but related movements began to build steam in the 1970s and '80s, and by the 1990s, researchers realized that a lot of people used alternative remedies either alone or in conjunction with Western medicine. In fact, the numbers were so high that universities like Harvard, Stanford, George Washington, and Yale began to study various forms of natural medicine and alternative therapies. And by 2000, hospitals and medical schools devised treatments using both complementary and alternative medicine because patients demanded these treatments alongside more traditional care.

5. Nature Is Medicine

The last key part in the evolution of our view of health and medicine is the growing awareness that prescription drugs aren't always the only answer or cure for much of what ails us. Many times, herbal and natural remedies are just as effective and are actually safer than some of the drugs we use. In fact, most drugs come from plants. Scientists find an active ingredient in a plant that has a particular pharmacological effect in the healing process. A pharmaceutical company then isolates it, makes it synthetically, magnifies its power, and packages it into a pill. Aspirin, for example, is a derivative of white willow bark and its active ingredient is salicylic acid. Taken in large amounts, aspirin can cause internal bleeding, but if you were to take the white willow bark in its whole plant form, its other ingredients would counteract the side effects of the salicylic acid.

> "With R.E.M. we were, I guess, at the forefront of the Green Tour Movement, trying to make less of a footprint. It always feels good to make a statement. My feeling about environmental activism has always been that everyone should do it on the level at which they're comfortable. Do what makes you feel good yet still able to perform the best you can."
>
> —MIKE MILLS, SONGWRITER, BASSIST, KEYBOARDIST, R.E.M.

CHANGING PARADIGMS IN FOOD

As revolutions brewed in health care, our understanding of the impact of food on our health evolved concomitantly, including three major paradigm shifts:

1. Food Is Medicine

The old way of thinking saw food only as a source of energy. Diets revolved entirely around calories—if you wanted to lose weight, you were given a calorie allotment. Fat, carbohydrates, and protein could be measured in energy, so it didn't matter *what* you ate, only the number of calories the food contained. Today we understand that our food is composed of a variety of macronutrients and micronutrients, all of which our body needs in different quantities—what we eat matters vitally. Diet can treat, manage, or reverse some of the chronic disease conditions in which pharmacological interventions were used in the past. For example, blueberries contain antioxidants called *anthocyanins* that lower blood sugar, which makes them a beneficial food for people with diabetes. This idea works both ways: some food components have the power to stave off or heal disease, while others can cause disease. This way of thinking further bolstered the organic food movement, because consumers believe that food grown without harmful poisons has fewer toxins for the body to clean and more nutritional value.

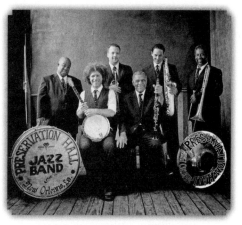

PRESERVATION HALL JAZZ BAND
(DANNY CLINCH)

"You have to think like 'Food Is Medicine.' If the doctor prescribes some medicine for your heart that you have to take three times per day, then you better believe that I am going to take that pill three times per day. Food should be no different. There are certain things that you just need to eat every day."

—BEN JAFFE, BANDLEADER, UPRIGHT BASS AND TUBA PLAYER,

PRESERVATION HALL JAZZ BAND

2. Food Is Information

The Human Genome Project spurred the development of a new science, called *nutrigenomics*, based on the concept that nutrition also affects our genes. The idea is that nutrients and phytochemicals in foods provide different information to our genes that affects our bodies in both good and bad ways. This information can change the way our genes and cells express themselves. Healthier foods lead to healthier cells and gene expression, while toxic foods cause degeneration and disease. This means that, rather than being stuck with the DNA blueprint we're born with, we can improve our genetic outcome by choosing the right foods, like fresh organic produce rather than processed, prepackaged items.

This once-alternative concept, now mainstream, has spurred the growth of health food markets, organic and vegetarian restaurants, and menus filled with local, seasonal, and organic ingredients.

3. The Slow Food Movement

A new way of looking at food that developed out of France and Italy, the Slow Food movement began in 1989 as a rebellion against fast-food culture. The "Slow Food" way of thinking challenges us all to take into account the culture and customs of what we eat, where it's sourced, and how it's harvested. The idea is that food should be celebrated, not packaged or heavily preserved so it stays on shelves for years without going bad, then gulped down while in the car. When people take the time to experience healthy food and what it really tastes like, they enjoy it. The cultural celebration of food and its cultivation is at the forefront of the Slow Food movement.

TALKIN' 'BOUT A REVOLUTION

The revolutionary philosophies brewing in health and nutrition paralleled what was happening during the same time period in music. Rock & roll began with the blues in the 1950s. The music was innovative and rebellious. In the '60s and '70s, rock & roll artists began to see that they served as a voice for social and political causes. This was very distinct from the mass appeal of mainstream pop culture and music. The "peace and love" counterculture also reflected a return to nature with an emphasis on health and spiritual awareness.

The movement gained momentum, and through the '70s, '80s, and '90s, rock & roll developed into different genres. Each one spawned a specific style, culture, and fashion to go with it. In the late '80s and early '90s, the alternative rock movement grew with bands such as R.E.M., Nirvana, and Pearl Jam, who were considered "alternative" because they weren't played on mainstream radio. They were first featured on college stations, but then exploded onto mainstream radio in the mid-'90s, at about the same time that alternative medicine became popular.

There are a lot of parallels between the rise of alternative health and music. What was once considered fringe thinking was suddenly more widely accepted. "Alternative" evolved to become mainstream.

By the late '90s and early 2000s, alternative health practices had become widely accepted. Rock stars began to understand their influence on culture more fully and began using their voices and music not only to express themselves, but also embrace the social responsibility that comes with being an artist. Different causes were born, such as the green movement, green festivals and tours, and charity and benefit concerts, such as the Tibetan Freedom Concert, Farm Aid, and Live Aid.

The synchronicity in the consciousness of medicine and music makes sense. Artists are natural messengers for alternative ideas and actions because they generally are sensitive, creative, and in tune with humanity. They realize the impact they have on people and want to use that power to make the world a better place. This is not unlike the many health-care practitioners today who are seeking alternatives to the monumental challenges. It's difficult to ignore that kind of authenticity. For this reason, rock stars make incredible ambassadors for health.

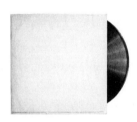

BONUS TRACKS

"I don't eat any fast food ever. I have not in twenty-five to thirty years. I eat only organic fresh foods, meats, vegetables, and fruits. I will do this till I die. It is in my DNA and what I am as a human, so I have learned to do it right, and now it is as much for fun and I am a hell of a lot healthier."

—STEVE LUKATHER, GUITARIST, TOTO

"I don't think in terms of alternative. It's just a way of life, always learning, gaining insight. I have at various times worked with all forms of body healers—no fasts, no detoxes, just mindful living."

–IAN ASTBURY, SINGER, SONGWRITER, THE CULT

"I don't believe in magic or witchcraft. I don't light candles to change my fate. I'm not into patchouli oil or the Grateful Dead. I don't believe in numerology, astrology, or tarot cards. However, I do believe that natural medicine is a very logical and relevant part of modern medicine. To ignore it in favor of the limited and often myopic approach of profit-driven insurance, pharmaceutical, and hospital industries is a mistake. I'm not saying traditional drugs and surgery are unnecessary. I'm simply saying they should be some of many tools that live on the more extreme side of a toolbox full of options that include much more preventative and natural approaches."

—GABRIEL ROTH (AKA BOSCO MANN), BASSIST AND SONGWRITER,

SHARON JONES & THE DAP-KINGS

"The weird thing about traveling with French people was that they always, no matter how little time they had, they always insisted on stopping for a meal. We never once went to a café or a rest stop or a gas station. We would pull in at a restaurant, they would sit down, and they put the f@%-ing napkin on their laps. They have a glass of wine and use a knife and fork. And they have a little conversation and a three-course meal! They work to live. They don't live to work like we do here."

—ANGELA McCLUSKEY, SINGER, SONGWRITER,

TELEPOP, WILD COLONIALS

"Armenians historically have had a lot of art and music in our blood. I am lucky to have been given the opportunity to speak universal truths through the arts."

—SERJ TANKIAN, SINGER, SONGWRITER, COMPOSER,

MULTI-INSTRUMENTALIST, RECORD PRODUCER, POET,

AND POLITICAL ACTIVIST, SYSTEM OF A DOWN

"I'm very aware of politics and the environment. Pollution is with us now forever. If I was president, the first thing I would do is clean up the plastic island the size of Texas floating in the ocean, and solar power would be mandatory. Eat organic!"

—JOHN WAITE, SINGER, SONGWRITER

"There is currently a paradigm shift toward sustainability and environmentalism that is happening in all aspects of society. . . . Lifestyle, culture, industry, health, food, fashion, consumerism, and media. Music, art, food, fashion, and film all have an aesthetic quality. Things that are beautiful and natural are healthier. Just as things that are natural and healthy are inherently more beautiful. The consumer is ultimately going to drive the paradigm shift to a healthier and happier world."

—ADRIAN GRENIER, MUSICIAN, ACTOR

"I worked with Paul McCartney in 2013 on his album *New*. He keeps his sessions vegetarian (and gangster). I felt so good that I ended up going vegetarian for half a year. I didn't stick with it (I hope Sir Paul is not reading this), but I've definitely tempered my diet considerably. I try to eat regularly, but I'm also a big fan of the late diner. Although I'm smart enough to know now that eating an ice cream sundae at 1 a.m. is guaranteed to bring on scarily lucid dreams of the zombie apocalypse."

—MARK RONSON, PRODUCER, ARTIST, DJ,
AMY WINEHOUSE, LILY ALLEN, BRUNO MARS,
AND **SIR PAUL McCARTNEY**

THE ROCKSTAR REMEDY

CHAPTER 3

TOTAL HEALTH TRANSFORMATION IN FIVE STAGES

When was the last time you were hanging out with friends, sipping green shakes, and talking about how cool it is to be healthy? Probably not recently, or maybe not ever. That's because most people think great health kills the fun and joy of living. But it's the opposite. You become more vibrant and joyful when you feel good and are *balanced* in mind, body, and spirit. If rock stars, the kings and queens of cool, are using natural medicine and alternative treatments to help them live life to the fullest while taking care of their bodies at the same time, you can, too. It's my mission to show you that it's cool to be healthy, and that great health will improve the quality and enjoyment of your life. My program—grounded in the principles discussed in this chapter—has been tested for two decades on the most extreme lifestyles in the world. The result is a proven plan that guarantees true transformation that lasts a lifetime.

The first step, the one you can do right now, is to ask yourself: "If anything were possible, how would I want to live my life?" I want you to really think about what your best possible life would look like, and the kinds of activities, habits, and relationships that would populate that life. Now I want you to think about your health. What would your health look like in that ideal life? How close or far is it from your current state of health? How does your current state of health help or prevent you from having that ideal life? The truth is, if we don't have our health, we don't have anything. So the first step toward living a better life is to create better health.

HEALTH IS ABOUT MORE THAN YOUR BODY

When I say that I want you to think about your "health," I don't just mean that I want you to think about your blood pressure. A holistic assessment of your life is the only way to really know what's going on with your body. In fact, your emotional and spiritual state—how stressed or anxious or happy you are—can be just as important to the state of your overall health as what's indicated in lab reports and blood tests. Think about your goals for your health—do they include how you feel, mentally? True health is a state of harmony in body, mind, and spirit within the context of your social system and environment. My job is to help you shift your thinking about health beyond your physical state.

The words "health" and "healthy" are thrown around a lot these days, and sometimes their meaning becomes a little cloudy. So let's take a closer look at what "health" really means.

- **HEALTH IS A PILGRIMAGE, NOT A DESTINATION.** Health is not a place where you arrive and your life magically becomes perfect and you'll never have to do anything to maintain it. Sometimes everything seems to be great. Other times, you run into obstacles. These obstacles are opportunities to transform your life. Often the negative experiences have more transformative power than the positive ones because they are opportunities to reevaluate your situation, determine what's important, and move in a new direction.

- **HEALTH IS ABOUT DIFFERENT KINDS OF BALANCE.** A balanced lifestyle is different for each person. For some of you, it's a daily health regime with specific rituals that spread balance throughout the day. If you're in this group, you likely have a little bit of fun every day, some exercise, some healthy food, but the routine doesn't change that much. For others (like many of my clients), your rhythm is on a pendulum where the extremes last weeks at a time, where you're completely immersed in working to meet a deadline or playing during a holiday and then, when that cycle slows down, you enjoy a long period of time dedicated to maintaining healthy habits. You detox, rejuvenate, and reconnect with family and friends. One thing rock stars have taught me is that you can't judge anyone's approach as wrong. Not everyone can be balanced every day.

"Eating a balanced diet in New Orleans is an incredible challenge. My town is historically not healthy for you. Eating in New Orleans is an event in itself. A lunch can be three hours long. That's part of the joy of New Orleans. Everything is a celebration!"

—BEN JAFFE, BANDLEADER, UPRIGHT BASS AND TUBA PLAYER,
PRESERVATION HALL JAZZ BAND

- **HEALTH IS AN ADVENTURE.** Life is a celebration! My philosophy is what you do for your health must fit into your lifestyle and be enjoyable, rather than isolating or extreme. I encourage you to celebrate your life through social activities and fun experiences that can be woven into a health regime. If you like to dance, take a dance class. If you love to swim, go to the pool. And if you're most yourself when socializing, enjoy dinners out where you can eat a variety of foods and enjoy an antioxidant-boosting glass of red wine. Doing what you love becomes a motivator that inspires your journey.

"My whole focus now is to be as healthy and as good of a dad as I can possibly be. I see a lot of my friends who are in really bad shape, either because of substances or physically they're just way out of shape—they can't even run in the backyard with their kids, let alone go snowboarding or surfing. I'm gonna do all that stuff! Can't wait. This winter, we're getting our son, Revel, on skis. I was just in Hawaii for a week, and I was in the ocean with Revel, four hours a day. I want to be seventy and still be able to ride a snowboard when my son is twenty-two. Everything I do is about longevity and remaining fit and healthy because I want to be there. For him."

—SCOTT IAN, FOUNDING GUITARIST, **ANTHRAX**

The key is to take steps to manage your health no matter where you are in your life at this very moment. My program doesn't promise "perfect health," an illusive idea that is impractical and unattainable for most of us, including celebrities. My plan is simply designed to take your dreams and stretch them a little further. What small, but life-changing, shifts can you make in how you live to move you toward greater vitality, happiness, and longevity?

Life is your stage. Are you ready to live like a rock star?

FIVE STAGES OF RxSTAR TRANSFORMATION

Most of my regular clients experience the same pendulum swing in lifestyle as my rock star clients: they're overextended, working on other people's schedules, experiencing insomnia, eating poorly if at all, skipping exercise, and feeling anxious and overwhelmed by the demands on their time. I see the same scenarios play out over and over where patients tell me that they're planning to spend the next few weeks working fourteen hours a day to meet a deadline. Then when they're done, they'll go back to exercising and eating right. It's their version of being on tour. During that time, my treatments for them are focused on harm reduction—supporting their bodies through the intensity and giving them the fuel they need to keep moving. It's during the downtime between huge projects that we're able to come back into balance.

"Never know what's coming. Tomorrow your doctor could tell you that you've got cancer and four months to live. That's the world. Thing about life that's sad but true is we get too soon old and too late smart. And smart means that you wake up and look at things before they pass you by. Every one of us goes through it. I started to see it when I was fifty. They don't write that into your birth certificate.

It should be written in: DON'T DO WHAT EVERYONE DOES. Don't find out too late about your ailment or disease when you could have done something about it."

—STEVEN TYLER, SINGER, SONGWRITER, MULTI-INSTRUMENTALIST, **AEROSMITH**

No matter where you currently are on the spectrum of health, there are five key areas of transformation in this program that will help you shift into the healthy zone.

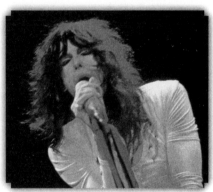

STEVEN TYLER
(MICK ROCK)

- STAGE 1: THE RxSTAR DETOX—DETOX IS THE TIME TO LET GO OF THINGS THAT DON'T SERVE YOU PHYSI-CALLY, MENTALLY, OR EMO-TIONALLY. I'll show you how to clear out all the things holding you back and create a clean slate, which opens up space for big transformations. What's different about my approach? Balance. This detox meets you where you are and fits around your lifestyle so you succeed in reaching your health goals. I'll give you two levels (moderate, or VIP, and strict, or Backstage) to choose from plus a variety of Harm Reduction Techniques to keep you on track.

- STAGE 2: FOOD—YOU WILL LEARN WHAT FOODS FUEL YOUR PERFORMANCE AND HOW TO INDULGE IN BALANCE. I'll show you what to eat for optimal looks, stamina, and focus. This same diet will enhance your energy levels, strengthen your immune system, and increase your vitality. You'll get grocery lists, best and worst nutrition options, ingredient substitutions, disease-fighting foods, and toxins to avoid. I'll even teach you how to make shopping, cooking, and meal planning an adventure, so you're motivated to try a whole new way of eating. And you will learn to appreciate that food is our greatest medicine.

- **STAGE 3: BODY—EXERCISE, LIKE DIET, CAN IMPROVE BEAUTY, PERFORMANCE, AND LONGEVITY.** But because your days are already a grind with work and family commitments, you have to love your exercise program or you won't do it. I'll give you ways to customize your workouts so they're fun and complement your lifestyle. I'll also teach you the regimens that rock stars follow both on and off tour every day to keep their bodies fit, functional, and youthful. After all, if you want to be your best night after night, you've got to move it.

- **STAGE 4: MIND AND SPIRIT—WE WILL LOOK AT HOW YOUR THOUGHTS, BELIEFS, EMOTIONS, AND ENVIRONMENT IMPACT EVERY CELL IN YOUR BODY AND MAKE A DIFFERENCE IN WHO YOU BECOME.** You'll examine and mend your relationships, build stronger connections with people you love, and let go of situations that don't enhance your journey. I'll give you strategies I teach my clients, such as meditation, mindfulness, spirituality, and prayer, to stay focused, positive, and empowered during their most stressful times. I'll share tips for managing challenging relationships, a common issue on rock tours and in the real world. One group I toured with had great creative chemistry and seemed to be so happy together onstage.

But in reality they disliked each other so much that they spent nearly seven thousand dollars a day on limos so that they could all ride separately from the hotel to the concert venue. I taught them, and will show you, more practical and cost-effective ways to resolve personal conflicts.

- **STAGE 5: SOCIALIZE—LIFE IS A PARTY.** It's normal to overindulge in alcohol, junk food, cigarettes, and other vices. The focus in this section is on treatments and therapies that bring your body chemistry, blood sugar levels, and outside pressures back into harmony so you can enjoy life without harming your health. I'll share tips on navigating social situations so you can have fun and connect with friends without sabotaging all the good habits you've already put in place.

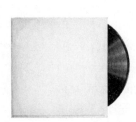

BONUS TRACKS

"Bono, man, that dude is like singing an opera concert and doing a marathon at the same time. He has the stamina of an Olympic athlete. On tour they play four or five marathons per week. I get tired just watching him!"

—MARK BATSON, PRODUCER, SONGWRITER,
ALICIA KEYS, DAVE MATTHEWS, EMINEM

"When I'm on the road, I try to be very careful with what I eat. Sometimes I'll fast the day of a show. It helps me get to the mental place that I want to be in while I'm playing. I'll usually get massages before or after a show. With Guns N' Roses, we play anywhere from two and a half hours to three and a half hours a night. It's like running a marathon!"

—RICHARD FORTUS, GUITARIST, GUNS N' ROSES

"The most important thing for health and longevity while touring is to be with friends that you love and trust like family. We are now over thirty and been through the shit and the fighting. Laughing and having fun with these friends is like a surf camp or vacation. We have become very healthy because we all have babies that are two to four years old. Now we all sit around and show pictures of our kids, not hot chicks. We show videos of funny things our kids do."

—ORI KAPLAN, SAXOPHONIST, BALKAN BEAT BOX

"My favorite healthy recipe? Don't smoke, anything. No drugs. Easy on the drink. Eat a balanced diet with friends whenever possible. Avoid crazy health fads. Don't drink and drive. Don't walk and text. Be a good person."

—JOE SATRIANI, GUITARIST

"I feel that talking about the disease lessened its power over me, and hopefully it helps others do the same. There is a form of healing that comes from both sharing my personal experiences and ideas and hearing other people tell me theirs. For me, the CCFA played the biggest role in my opening up and telling my story, and everything got better for me and my health after that happened. There is a camp called Camp Oasis, where kids with Crohn's and ulcerative colitis can go and feel 'normal.' I support the Northwest Chapter Camp Oasis program with a yearly benefit concert called Flight to Mars. My message is that the less you isolate yourself, the more you open doors to the life you want to live. These diseases can make a person want to hide away and be alone, and I get that, but it only keeps you from all the connections you need, and all the great things you want to accomplish. It's important to open up and talk to others who are dealing with similar issues so you can watch and learn how they are dealing with it. The power in that is immense!"

—MIKE McCREADY, GUITARIST, VOCALS,

SONGWRITER, **PEARL JAM**

"A lot of people believe that there is a finish line or destination where all our self-doubt will be extinguished. And when we hit that and we we're not fixed we say to ourselves, 'Oh, shit, now what do I do?' I am no stranger to that. I had to do a lot of work. Still do."

—DAVE NAVARRO, **JANE'S ADDICTION**

PART TWO

STAGE ONE: THE RxSTAR DETOX: START WITH A CLEAN SLATE

CHAPTER 4

DETOX 101

For many of us, loving life tends to include a lot more indulgence than deprivation. When you fill your life (or your plate or your glass) with what you love, it's important to have a program that you complete periodically to ensure all this fun adds years to your life, instead of taking them away. That's the pendulum on the health spectrum swinging you back toward vibrancy, radiance, and longevity. That's the RxStar Detox.

Cleansing, however, isn't just for pizza lovers and beer drinkers. Most of us don't get as much sleep or eat as many greens or drink as much water as we should. Even if you're normally pretty healthy and rarely indulge to excess, the RxStar Detox is a great way to recalibrate your diet, nix any lingering unhealthy habits, reduce stress, and reignite your energy. I don't know about you, but reducing stress always sounds good to me!

When we detox, we give ourselves an opportunity to cleanse our lives of anything that isn't serving us in a positive way. What do these "things" look like? Bad bosses, vending machine diets, energy-draining friends, negative thoughts, self-defeating behaviors, skipping the gym. Once you recognize and release what's not working, you can rebuild and refine your health on a much stronger foundation. That's the gist of these next 21 days. Clearing out the bad to make way for the good. You're creating a beautiful blank canvas so your body can better absorb nutrients. That's not so scary, is it?

WHY DO I NEED TO DETOX?

This is a question many of my clients ask me. They've heard the term, but they're not sure what toxins are and how they got into their bodies in the first place. Let's take a closer look at why it's so important to detoxify your body on a regular basis.

"The human body never does more than it has to. It doesn't decide on its own to gain fat or lose weight—if it does in fact start doing stuff without external 'input,' such as food, drugs, or exercise, then it probably means you're sick. We're all equipped with internal voices and sensors that let us know how to keep ourselves 'in shape.' Just gotta stop talking (or thinking too loud) and listen."

—KANE ROBERTS, HEAVY METAL GUITARIST,
FORMERLY WITH ALICE COOPER (LF)

"Letting go of negative situations is hard for anyone. The good thing about being on tour is that you go to different places from day to day, which can cast a different mood on a situation. It's a great tool for moving on. You can say to yourself, 'This just happened here and I'm focusing on whatever is next.' You force yourself to let go of it."

—JULIA HALTIGAN, SINGER, SONGWRITER,
JULIA HALTIGAN & THE HOOLIGANS (SB)

There are two types of toxins: external toxins (exotoxins) and internal toxins (endotoxins). It is natural to have a certain amount of toxicity in our bodies. For example, the process of cellular respiration—the mechanism by which our cells produce energy—generates waste products that are considered "toxins" (endotoxins). It's not a big deal, because your body works to eliminate these toxins in the same way it eliminates any waste—via urine, bowel movements, and sweat. But when the amount of toxins inside the body is greater than what can be eliminated, an imbalance occurs. This can cause irritation or inflammation of the cells and tissues, which in turn causes organs and systems to malfunction. High toxicity may also result in unpleasant physical symptoms, such as feeling tired or unfocused or experiencing skin or digestive issues.

Endotoxins are generally the by-products of normal, everyday metabolic activities, but they can also result from negative and destructive thoughts, emotions, and stress. There are fleeting thoughts and then there are those bigger, all-consuming emotions you push aside. You think they're gone because you're not actively thinking about them, but in fact, they may be impacting your immune, digestive, and nervous systems. Stress, anxiety, and other negative emotions have a very real impact on your health, and so a key part of detoxing is not only nourishing the body, but also nourishing the mind.

WHAT CREATES ENDOTOXINS?

Anger and resentment

Anxiety

Bacterial end products

Bowel toxins

Fear

Free radicals
Hormones
Insecurity and self-criticism
Jealousy
Metabolic wastes
Pessimism

Exotoxins enter your body when you ingest them in food or drink, inhale them into your lungs, or make other physical contact with them. For example, secondhand smoke is an exotoxin, as are many of the chemicals and additives in food products. Emotionally, negative and unhealthy environments, activities, and relationships also fit the category of exotoxins.

WHAT CREATES EXOTOXINS?

Air pollution
Alcohol
Bacteria
Beauty and skin care products
Caffeine
Cleaning supplies
Drugs and medications
Environmental allergens
Food allergens
Food dyes
Food preservatives
Heavy metals

Hormones in animal products

Negative people

Negative relationships

Pesticides

Petroleum

Plastics

Poor working environments

Poverty

Smoking

Violent living conditions

Viruses

Water residues

GETTING RID OF THE TOXINS

Your body is an incredible work of mastery. It's designed with many systems—digestive, circulatory, respiratory, and more—that are constantly communicating and relating to each other, with the nervous system running the entire show.

There are seven systems that help eliminate and cleanse toxins from your body. Think of them like your very own team of personal assistants. They work behind the scenes 24/7 (yes, even while you sleep) to help you maintain optimal health and a disease-free state.

"I have Gilbert's syndrome. I was hospitalized in my early twenties and very jaundiced and sick. I've always had to watch what I eat and maintain a balance. That condition, to some degree, has moderated my rock & roll lifestyle and probably saved me on many occasions from

A detox or cleanse is like giving these systems some much-needed support so they can continue to sweep toxins from your body. Your system can get pretty overwhelmed from the simple act of living in a modern world with processed foods, stress, pollution, and a demanding lifestyle. This can cause cell damage, then tissue damage, and eventually it can lead to disease. Detoxing helps to improve the function of the organs that remove unwanted invaders from our bodies so that they can do their job more efficiently.

The main focus of my detox is to treat the liver and the gut. I've learned that if I focus on detoxing these two systems in a new patient, we're usually able to resolve 50 to 90 percent of the symptoms he or she came in with. From there, I have a clean slate to move to the next phase of healing, which is typically rebuilding.

There are seven major systems involved in detoxification:

1. Lungs and Respiratory System

When you inhale, your lungs reoxygenate your blood and circulate this freshly oxygenated blood to fuel the heart, the arteries, and finally the entire body. When you exhale, these same organs expel toxic waste, aka carbon dioxide.

This process makes the lungs ground zero for airborne toxins, chemicals, viruses, bacteria, and allergens. Luckily, detoxification is as simple as, well, breathing. If you're like most people, you tend to take shallow breaths, especially in tense or stressful situations. In fact, most of us take in just enough air to stay alive. The more deeply you breathe, however, the more oxygen you deliver to every cell of your body.

2. Lymphatic System (Including the GALT)

The lymphatic system is a complex network of vessels, nodes, and pathways that carry lymphatic fluid throughout the body, much the way arteries and veins circulate blood. In fact, lymphatic vessels flow alongside your blood vessels. Unlike the circulatory system, the lymphatic system does not have a pump (the heart). Instead it relies on muscle movement and contraction to push fluid through its channels. This means exercise and massage aren't just important for soothing your mind and muscles; they're also essential for a healthy lymphatic system.

Lymphatic fluid carries white blood cells called lymphocytes. These cells act like bodyguards, disabling harmful foreign invaders picked up from your blood. Ever notice that when you're sick, your lymph nodes are swollen? That's because they are working overtime to rid your body of foreign invaders.

Your GALT is also part of the lymphatic system. The GALT is the intersection of our gastrointestinal system, immune system, and nervous system and is made up of a network of immune cells and membranes that line the inside passages of our body. Think of it as our "inside skin." The functions of the skin are to absorb nutrients and provide a barrier that protects toxins from getting into the body. In a sense, it's part of our immune system. The GALT works similarly, but it lines the inside passages of our body, including the sinuses, nose, lungs, mouth, esophagus, stomach, large intestine, small intestine, colon, vagina, urethra, and bladder.

- **A HEALTHY GALT ABSORBS NUTRIENTS AND ELIMINATES TOXINS.**
  When we eat, foods—protein, fat, and carbohydrates—get

broken down by enzymes in the stomach and small intestine into smaller units. Protein turns into amino acids, fat into fatty acids, and carbohydrates into glucose. These micronutrients transport across the GALT layer into the bloodstream and then out to the proper tissues.

- **TOXINS, WASTE, AND UNDIGESTED FOOD CAN'T MAKE THEIR WAY THROUGH THE GALT SO THEY GET ELIMINATED THROUGH THE LARGE INTESTINE AS STOOL.** When the GALT does what it's supposed to do, nutrients get to your cells and waste goes straight to the exit. But if your GALT is weak, it doesn't matter how much green juice you drink—very few of the nutrients you're consuming are being absorbed by your body. Instead they pass right through like water. It's what I call "expensive urine."

- **THE GALT'S SECOND JOB IS TO PREVENT INFECTION.** When your GALT is healthy, you're less likely to get sick. You've probably seen this concept in action at the office. One person comes down with the flu. Half the office soon catches it, while the other half isn't affected at all. People who get sick aren't breathing more bugs than the others. Much of their immunity depends on the health of their GALT.

When the GALT is weakened, fewer nutrients are absorbed and risk of infection increases as more toxins and allergens are able to make their way into our bloodstream.

When more toxins enter your bloodstream, white blood cells—the antibodies programmed to recognize what belongs in your body and what doesn't—flag them as foreign invaders they need to get rid of and produce an immune or allergy response. Most allergies and immune problems start with a breakdown of the GALT.

WHAT IS LEAKY GUT SYNDROME?

"Leaky gut syndrome" is the degeneration or breakdown of the GALT. It's a bit of a misnomer because it affects not just the stomach wall but also the entire GALT lining in the respiratory, digestive, urinary, and reproductive systems. What would cause this breakdown of the GALT? Medicines such as antibiotics, steroids, pain medicine, birth control pills; lifestyle factors including stress, recreational drugs, and alcohol; and food sources such as sugar, caffeine, artificial sweeteners, and food additives. The list goes on and on. Modern life can challenge our GALT. Stress speeds this process because it releases a hormone called cortisol, which also weakens this lining.

Leaky gut is tough to diagnose and many conventional practitioners question its validity. That said, if you experience several of the symptoms below, I suggest you see your doctor. There's a chance that leaky gut syndrome could be undermining your immunity and your overall health.

- Frequent respiratory conditions like colds, flu, allergies, sinus, asthma, bronchitis, and more
- Persistent digestive problems like gas, bloating, constipation, sensitivity and intolerance to foods, diarrhea, nausea, irritable bowel syndrome, heartburn, and acid reflux
- Skin conditions like rashes, eczema, acne, and psoriasis
- Urinary tract infections
- Reproductive organ infections such as herpes, yeast infections, and human papillomavirus (HPV)
- Fatigue, malaise, brain fog, and headaches

Leaky gut syndrome is also linked to an increased chance of developing an autoimmune disease or general inflammation in the body. When GALT breakdown is at a late stage, you may experience many or all of these issues at some point. Most of us have some of these symptoms simply because we're living in modern times.

3. Kidneys and Urinary Tract

Many waste materials pass through your kidneys to be filtered and excreted through your bladder. What you eat and drink affects the health and functioning of your kidneys. Overloading them with animal products, sodium, refined sugar, processed foods, and alcohol can overtax them and impair functioning. They're also sensitive to heavy metals like lead and mercury. Similar to the colon detoxification system, when you don't drink adequate amounts of water or urinate frequently enough, your urine passed will have a more pungent odor and darker color. That's because it contains a concentrated amount of waste.

4. Circulatory System

Your blood is the vital fluid pumped from your heart to your organs and cells through an arterial network. Your veins carry blood to your heart and from there it is pumped to the lungs, where it is exchanged for fresh oxygen and nutrients and then recycled again.

5. Skin

Your skin is the first line of defense against organisms and toxins entering the body. It is also the place where vitamin D gets activated by exposure to sunlight. The blood directly feeds the skin; therefore toxins in the blood are eliminated through the skin. This is why toxicity can lead to acne, rashes, hives, eczema, and psoriasis.

6. Large Intestine and Colon

This is the last segment of the gut. Toxins are dumped into the colon via the liver, gallbladder, and the lymphatic system. They are then eliminated out of the body. When waste isn't eliminated efficiently, toxic bowel may result.

7. Liver

If you're living large, it's likely your liver is taking a beating. The liver detoxifies through a network of enzymes. The role of the liver enzymes is to convert fat-soluble toxins into water-soluble substances so that they can be eliminated through the kidneys and intestines. Think of the liver as the superhero of detoxification—it neutralizes a large number of internal and external pollutants. In other words, it makes toxins less toxic.

Your liver is always on the clock. If you have a weak GALT, there is more burden on the liver since toxins that make their way into the blood will have to get filtered through the liver again. Liver detoxification occurs in two stages of enzymatic processes. In order for these enzymatic processes to work properly, the liver needs numerous vitamins, minerals, and amino acids. No nutrients? No detox. That means if you're fasting—going eight or more hours without eating—your liver slows down.

The liver rids your body of toxins in two phases. In phase 1, a toxin is broken down into an intermediate compound that is often more toxic than the original substance because it is less chemically stable. In phase 2, enzymes bind or conjugate to this toxin and make it water-soluble so it's easily excreted out of the body.

The RxStar Remedy Detox supports these seven systems so that they work more efficiently to help your body eliminate waste and by-products of your diet and lifestyle. They are the watchdogs that keep you balanced physiologically. The supplements, shakes, food plan, and therapies listed in this chapter are designed to support your body in moving toxins out while you change your lifestyle to prevent toxins from coming in. This combined strategy makes my approach safe and simple to do, no matter how crazy life gets.

It's important to note that when detoxing is done properly, it shouldn't make you sick. If you get ill when you're cleansing, this isn't a "healthy" or "healing" reaction, as was once thought. Instead, one of two things may be happening:

1. You're fasting or not getting the nutrients you need for the liver to work properly. When you fast, your liver pathways slow down, which increases free radicals in the blood. There aren't enough nutrients to create the enzymes necessary to move the toxins out of your body.

2. You're ignoring your GALT. Many modern cleanses involve purging and flushing the liver rapidly. This causes toxins to move out quickly, but if your GALT is weak, or if you have leaky gut syndrome, the toxins get reabsorbed back into the bloodstream, causing illness.

Therefore, a detox regime that supports the liver and gut/GALT should result in an improvement in symptoms without making you feel worse.

WHAT'S IN IT FOR YOU?

Fantastic health! The benefits of detoxification are as personal to you as your habits and lifestyle. That's what makes detoxing so rewarding and effective. You may choose to detox seasonally or yearly or whenever you're feeling like you could use a little more vitality. The more regularly you cleanse—and incorporate the detox mind-set into daily living—the greater and more lasting the results. And the more exciting the adventure!

Benefits of the RxStar Remedy Detox:

- REDUCED CRAVINGS FOR SUGAR, CAFFEINE, NICOTINE, ALCOHOL, DRUGS
- INCREASED ENERGY
- INCREASED MENTAL CLARITY
- RESET EATING HABITS
- WEIGHT LOSS
- IMPROVED ABSORPTION OF NUTRIENTS
- ELIMINATES TOXINS
- FACILITATES HEALTHY ORGAN FUNCTIONS
- IMPROVED DIGESTION
- STRENGTHENED IMMUNE SYSTEM
- CLEARER SKIN
- LESS STRESS, ANXIETY, AND DEPRESSION
- ENHANCED SPIRITUAL AWARENESS

- INCREASED VITALITY
- STRENGTHENED WILLPOWER AND SENSE OF ACCOMPLISHMENT
- HELPS RELEASE NEGATIVE EMOTIONS AND THOUGHTS

YOUR BODY IS A METAPHOR

Your physical body is a metaphor that can tell you a lot about what is happening in your life emotionally and spiritually. For example, if someone has an autoimmune disease, such as rheumatoid arthritis, that person's immune system is attacking her body, destroying her connective tissue and joints. What story is her body telling? She may discover she's self-critical, judgmental, or even a perfectionist. Her body's assault on itself may be, in part, a manifestation of her emotions within her cells.

> "I just tried [a three-day detox cleanse] and man! Day four was epic . . . I wore a bright yellow shirt! I never wear bright happy colors. The shirt resembled how I felt!! Like the sun!"
>
> —TOMMY LEE, FOUNDING DRUMMER, MÖTLEY CRÜE AND METHODS OF MAYHEM

This same metaphor can also be used for healing. A good detox program rids your body, as well as your emotions, spirit, and lifestyle, of what doesn't serve it. This is the perfect opportunity to release resentments, resolve situations, and stop engaging in negative thought patterns or habits that are no longer useful in your life. It is also a great time to clean the house and closets and get organized.

During this three-week program, consider everything in your world that's holding you back from your greatness and identify what you're no longer willing to accept or live with. Post-detox, you will rejuvenate and rebuild your body. At the same time, this is an opportunity to bring in new experiences, healed relationships, and healthy habits.

While the detox focuses on letting go and creating space, the post-detox phase will give you the clarity, drive, and platform to integrate everything you want physically, emotionally, spiritually, and socially.

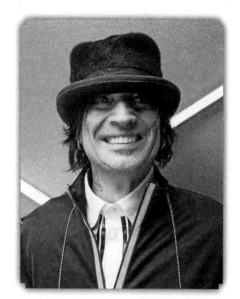

TOMMY LEEE
(MICK ROCK)

FOUR PHASES OF THE RxSTAR REMEDY DETOX

The key to success in any detox is to *first* remove what's not working in your life and *then* build and refine your health from a fresh start. Imagine that the four phases are like your favorite band. They all need to work synergistically to create the perfect sound. Sure, you still hear music when one member of the band is not present, but it's not the full effect. The same thing happens with this detox. Extraordinary results can occur when you're holistically cleansing *all* areas of your life. Is a little better than nothing? Absolutely. Like everything in this book, detox is centered on balance. But the more positive steps you take for your health, the more profound your results at the end of 21 days.

This isn't one of those "live a crazy party life all the time and purify yourself once a year" programs that will help you for a month but do nothing to improve your life long-term. My goal is not to give you some fashionable or trendy plan so you can go back to polluting yourself afterward. If you make these changes and stick with them 90 percent of the time, you'll live a longer, happier, healthier life because you'll be consistent. When you do veer off the path the other 10 percent of the time, go back to a strict detox to rid your body of any accumulated toxins and support your immune system. There are four phases to the detox.

Phase 1: Detox Your Diet

The core of the detox is diet. You'll find that you make more conscious choices about what you eat as you gain more clarity, focus, and energy. The goal is to detox your body from the inside, starting with what and how you eat. This includes:

- A TWENTY-ONE-DAY EATING PLAN BASED ON CLEAN FOODS THAT REGULATE BLOOD SUGAR AND BALANCE HORMONES.
- THE RxSTAR DETOX SHAKE AS A BREAKFAST AND/OR LUNCH REPLACEMENT. This delicious shake is packed with nutrients that support the liver, kidneys, GALT, and intestines.
- VITAMIN- AND MINERAL-BASED SUPPLEMENTS THAT MOVE YOU TOWARD BALANCE AND SUPPORT THE SEVEN SYSTEMS THAT KEEP YOU HEALTHY.

- ORGANIC HERBAL TEAS THAT ENHANCE THE DETOXIFICATION PROCESS, CURB CRAVINGS, BOOST ENERGY, AND DEEPEN SLEEP.
- CLEAN WATER TO FLUSH OUT TOXINS AND HYDRATE.

Phase 2: Detox Your Body

Exercise, body treatments, and healthy beauty regimens take detoxification to a deeper level by helping your system move out toxins through sweat. During cleansing, however, not all workouts are created equal. Because your body is already working extra hard during a cleanse, I've tailored specific moves and regimens designed for minimal impact and maximum results.

Phase 3: Detox Your Mind

No matter what type of changes you make in your eating habits, it's important to make sure they stick by getting your brain on board, too. For my Type A rock stars, this can often be the most challenging step. Addictions, stress, overwork, negativity, and relationship drama? I've seen it all. But at the end of the day, you answer to *you*—your mind, your body, your spirit.

Phase 4: Detox Your Home

Changes you make to your body on the inside need to be supported by your outside environment. Everything that contains toxins, including your lifestyle and home products, can be considered here. This is the time to clean house and create a healthy and nourishing living environment.

HOW TOXIC ARE YOU? THE DETOX QUIZ

Before you get started on the detox, I want you to take the quiz below, which will help you determine your toxicity levels and decide how to customize the detox for your individual needs and goals.

1. I have:
   A. done many detoxes and cleanses before with excellent results.
   B. done a detox before but have experienced negative symptoms.
   C. never done a detox or cleanse before.

2. My current health status is:
   A. good overall but I have minor problems.
   B. not great but I am not taking many medications.
   C. compromised and I am taking medications that are being monitored by a doctor.

3. I eat foods that are:
   A. primarily healthy and organic.
   B. well-rounded but not organic.
   C. mostly from restaurants, fast food, and packaged processed foods.

4. I grocery-shop at:
   A. natural food markets and farmer's markets.
   B. regular grocery stores.
   C. never shop or cook. I mostly eat out.

5. I am thinking about the next three weeks of my life, during which I will embark on the detox and:
    A. I have lots of downtime and time to implement the recommendations.
    B. I will be busy at work or at home and have little time to implement great changes.
    C. I will be traveling the entire time and living in hotel rooms.

6. Most of my meals are eaten at:
    A. home.
    B. a combination of home and in restaurants that have healthy options.
    C. In restaurants and from carry-outs that do not have the healthiest options.

7. I eat _____ meals per day.
    A. 3 to 4
    B. 1 to 2
    C. 1

8. I cannot do a detox unless it allows the following:
    A. chocolate
    B. coffee
    C. alcohol

9. My social life involves primarily:
    A. dinners with friends and hanging at home.
    B. dinners out with friends.
    C. drinking in bars with friends.

10. The idea of the detox sounds:
    A. exciting and easy for me.
    B. interesting but slightly intimidating.
    C. grueling and difficult.

If you answered (a) to more than seven questions, then you are a great candidate for the Backstage Cleanse.

The Backstage Cleanse recommendations are best suited for people who will have some downtime in the next three weeks. You live a fairly clean lifestyle and have most likely done a few detoxes in the past. You're pretty healthy already, but you're always looking for ways to improve and get healthier. This version of the detox is the strictest of the three, and includes a RxStar Detox Shake for breakfast.

If you answered (a) or (b) to more than seven questions, then you are a great candidate for the VIP Cleanse.

You want to get healthier but have limited time or opportunity to eat the way you'd prefer to eat. In fact, you may find yourself eating in restaurants for much of the cleanse. The recommendations for this level are tailored for people who are engaged in a very busy work life and have little downtime. You will focus on eating smaller meals throughout the day, starting with a RxStar Detox Shake for breakfast.

If you answered (c) to more than five questions, you are a Groupie.

The Groupies are people who are interested in the idea of detoxing and feeling better but they are under the care of a doctor for various conditions and may be taking several medications. If you are a Groupie, chances are you've never done a detox before.

If this is your first detox and you have a preexisting health condition, talk to your doctor about trying the nutritional component of the cleanse only. If your doctor approves, follow the food recommendations to the best of your ability. Do not take the RxStar Detox Shake unless it is approved by your doctor.

Remember, some effort is better than none when it comes to your health. If you hit a bump in the road or some aspect of the detox feels too restrictive, incorporate Harm Reduction Techniques and remind yourself that this is only 21 days. Once you get those under your belt, you will have moved the needle toward greater health and making healthy choices will take a lot less effort. But be honest with yourself, stay committed, and be accountable. Your health is worth it.

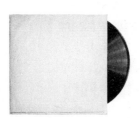

BONUS TRACKS

"I went gluten free a few years ago. Was always getting CT scans on my stomach for these abdominal pains that no doctor could figure out. They would do the tests, and the results were the same. 'You're clear.' But I was still having pains. Finally, a friend referred me to this doctor. He told me to try eliminating gluten from my diet. Literally, in two or three days, I was fine! My stomach never felt better."

—FRED COURY, DRUMMER, **CINDERELLA**

"I don't want to quit fun, either. You know? I'll quit drinking, and go on these cleanses and live clean, a couple months at a time. It usually has to be when I have nothing else going on. Health is such a weird thing. There are fads and trends. I've got a bunch of friends in LA now that are on this whole trip: it's called the 'bulletproof diet.' There is a lot of protein and not a lot of carbohydrates. But it's weird, man. They put butter in their coffee."

—CONOR OBERST, SINGER, SONGWRITER, GUITARIST,
BRIGHT EYES, LOS DESAPARECIDOS

"I really don't want to burn out, you know. I want to keep going and going as long as I can and in whatever form I have to adapt. The debts you incur as far as energy and health, those babies are hard to pay back. It is easy to burn the wick at both ends. The younger people are looking at me like, 'You eat like an old lady' or 'You eat this shit? Like an old man . . .' It is only because I have been through this stuff that I do this and because these are the priorities that keep you on tour."

—MIKE WATT, BASSIST,
MINUTEMEN, FIREHOSE, IGGY POP

CHAPTER 5

DETOX YOUR DIET

"Because I'm onstage and in fitted clothing all the time on the road, I lay off the sugary desserts, the complex carbs, and processed foods like pasta, potatoes, and bread. Of course, when I'm tired I crave sugar, so I don't have a hard fast rule on this, but I do my best to make it a lifestyle of eating low carb because I see instant results of a flatter stomach and a much leaner look."

—DAVE ELLEFSON, BASSIST AND FOUNDING MEMBER, MEGADETH

Here's the good news: this is not a starvation diet. No healthy cleanse should require you to severely restrict your calorie intake or deprive your body of the nourishment it needs to function properly.

This cleanse is designed to balance your hormones and blood sugar, which is essential to healthy weight, good energy, and an improved mood. Balancing blood sugar creates a steady flow of energy for the body to maintain all of its functions. If your blood sugar is low, your body goes into a crisis state, known as catabolism, during which it breaks down muscle, bone, and organ tissue to keep itself going. This in turn weakens all of your systems, promotes disease, and causes weight gain in the midsection. You might experience symptoms like fatigue, anxiety, mood swings, insomnia, and sugar cravings.

In order to restore balance to your blood sugar and hormones, we need to focus on your nutrition. If you are following the recommendations for the VIP or Backstage cleanse, you will start each day with a RxStar Detox Shake for breakfast that contains a minimum of 15 grams of protein. Then you'll eat several small meals throughout the day that consist of a combination of lean protein, healthy fats, and carbs. Always pair carbohydrates with lean protein to regulate blood sugar. This can be as simple as a handful of nuts with an apple or as well-rounded as wild-caught fish with a salad or whole grain.

What's the big deal about balancing sugar and hormones? Blood sugar balance involves regulation by two hormones—insulin and glucagon. Insulin is produced by the pancreas when carbohydrates are consumed. When you eat more carbs than your body can immediately burn, insulin signals the body to store the excess carbs as fat. Glucagon is produced by the liver when protein is consumed; it signals the body to tap into your fat reserve when extra energy is needed. Excess insulin production occurs when you eat a lot of carbohydrates without protein to balance it or when stress or addictions (such as caffeine, alcohol, and nicotine) cause your body to produce too much cortisol.

HARM REDUCTION TECHNIQUE: I WANT CANDY

Dried fruit should be considered a treat and eaten in moderation because its sugar content is highly concentrated and it often contains added sugars and sulfites. Basically, it's candy. A piece of dark chocolate made with 70 percent or greater cacao and organic sugars may be a better option.

Excess cortisol and insulin production, combined with the inability of your cells to use the insulin, may result in a condition known as insulin resistance. This can ultimately lead to a complex set of symptoms known as metabolic syndrome or syndrome X. Metabolic syndrome is one of the main sources of inflammation associated with most chronic diseases such as cancer, cardiovascular disease, diabetes, hormone imbalances, and obesity. This is why it's so essential to properly balance your blood sugar and, in turn, your hormones.

On the cleanse, we will accomplish this by eating:

- **FOODS THAT ENHANCE INSULIN FUNCTION,** such as organic fruits, vegetables, beans, nuts, seeds, whole grains, and flax and olive oils.
- **ORGANIC, WHOLE, UNPROCESSED FOODS**—in other words, clean foods—while avoiding or eliminating white flour, alcohol, sugar, caffeine, dairy, and hydrogenated fats.
- **GLUTEN-FREE GRAINS.** Gluten and gliadin—the main proteins in wheat and many grains—are the most common allergens in food. They're often the mystery substance triggering issues like fatigue, headaches, joint stiffness, irritable bowel syndrome, and bloating, along with more serious conditions like asthma, migraines, and autoimmune diseases. When you remove them from your diet, especially through a detox, often many undiagnosed symptoms disappear. Even when you're not cleansing, it's best to limit gluten-containing grains or products.

GLUTEN-FREE GETS A BAD RAP

If you've tried to navigate restaurant menus or food labels in an effort to avoid gluten, you know it can be tough. Many products contain gluten in minimal amounts; unless you are severely allergic, a minimum amount probably won't do much harm. It's more important to seek out the healthier, gluten-free alternatives for the main culprits: pastas, breads, crackers, muffins, and other baked goods.

Here are a few tips to make shopping for and ordering your dinner (and dessert!) a little easier:

Grains that contain gluten: barley, bulgur, durum, Kamut, rye, spelt, semolina, triticale, wheat
Gluten-free grains: amaranth, arrowroot, corn, kudzu, millet, oats, quinoa, rice

Your best bets for a gluten-*reduced* diet:

Breads: gluten-free labeled breads, sprouted grain breads, flatbreads, lavash, pita, tortillas
Cereals: granola, muesli, oats, rice
Cooked: brown rice, millet, quinoa
Crackers: rice, lentil, garbanzo bean
Pastas: corn, quinoa, rice, black bean
Flours: almond meal, soybean flour, cornmeal, arrowroot flour, tapioca starch flour

21 DAYS TO BETTER HEALTH

The RxStar Detox is simple. You'll start the day with a protein-rich shake. The RxStar Detox Shake is your "medicine"—it provides all the vitamins, minerals, and nutrients your body needs to recalibrate and eliminate toxins. Then you'll eat a clean lunch, dinner, and snacks. After tweaking your diet, you'll add in extra nutrition designed to support your detoxification and move you toward more balanced health.

This cleanse is extremely gentle because it's designed to support the liver, kidneys, and gastrointestinal organs *before* toxins are removed. This means that you should experience virtually no side effects other than what you might normally get from reducing caffeine or sugar intake if you're a heavy user.

See how simple it is? Again, it's all about balance. You can eat food. It will just be more nutritious food. You can eat at restaurants. They'll just be healthier restaurants and you'll make smarter menu choices. Happy hours, birthday parties, date nights. You can have it all without being the odd man out or harming your health.

Remember, the 21-day cleanse is broken down into two levels: the VIP Cleanse and the Backstage Cleanse. Use the results in the quiz from chapter 4 to determine where you should start. The goal is success, so choose the level that will work for you, your lifestyle, and your schedule. What you choose now might be different from what you choose the next time you do the detox.

H ere's a snapshot of the daily meal plan for the VIP and the Backstage levels. They're almost identical, except that with the more rigorous Backstage regimen, you can substitute a shake for a second meal.

VIP RxSTAR CLEANSE

BREAKFAST: RxStar Detox Shake
LUNCH: Clean meal
DINNER: Clean meal
SNACKS: Optional two with lean protein and healthy carbs

BACKSTAGE RxSTAR DETOX

BREAKFAST: RxStar Detox Shake
LUNCH: RxStar Detox Shake or clean meal
DINNER: Clean meal
SNACKS: Optional two with lean protein and healthy carbs

WHAT TO EAT

The chart below offers an overview of the foods allowed on the detox. It's a long and varied list—so you should never feel unsatisfied or hungry. When possible, always choose organic, unprocessed, locally grown, and all-natural varieties of recommended foods or ingredients.

The serving sizes are recommendations; the idea is that the smaller your portion sizes, the greater the variety of nutrients you will be able to eat every day. I don't expect you to count calories or weigh portions. Instead, I recommend eating a wide variety of foods from different categories so your body is nourished in the best possible way. Food is your medicine. When you give your body different options, you give it more tools for healing.

Note that the RxStar Detox does not include phases that involve eliminating or adding in food groups, supplements, or shakes. Many of my clients find phase-based programs confusing or too difficult to follow with a busy schedule. This cleanse is simple: You'll eat the foods listed below for snacks or meals every day in conjunction with the shakes and supplements. There are no calorie restrictions. Simply eat slowly, chew food well, and stop eating *before* you feel full. It takes time for your brain to recognize when it's satisfied, so the more slowly you eat, the less likely you are to overindulge.

After you complete the cleanse, follow the 90/10 Rule to keep the good nutrition you've just put into practice in check with real life.

RxStar Detox Shake

The RxStar Detox Shake is the star of both the VIP and Backstage cleanses. This recipe was designed to support the liver, kidneys, and gastrointestinal systems while providing a delicious breakfast meal replacement during your three-week cleanse. It's best as a meal replacement for breakfast, but if you're at the Backstage level and want faster results, you may also supplement with a shake for lunch.

The shake is delicious and takes just minutes to whip up. All you need is a blender and these six ingredients:

1. Functional Food Powder

First designed in the late '70s, functional foods are used today by medical and naturopathic doctors to affect a particular area of the metabolism. Look for hypoallergenic formulas with added multivitamins and at least 15 grams of rice, pea, or hemp protein. Functional food powders provide the nutrients necessary to support liver enzymes that gently and naturally filter toxins from the

DETOX FOODS

Food	Recommended VIP and Backstage	Avoid VIP and Backstage (moderate cleanse)	Avoid Backstage only (stricter cleanse)
Meat, Fish, Poultry, Eggs (2 to 3 servings of fish per week, 1 to 2 servings of chicken per week)	Organic chicken, turkey, fresh or canned wild-caught fish (anchovies, cod, flounder, halibut, mackerel, salmon, sardines, trout) Organic beef Organic lamb Wild game	Lunch meats, sausages, pork (yes, that means bacon), non-organic beef, non-organic chicken, shellfish, swordfish, farm-raised fish, egg substitutes, egg whites only VIP "cheat": Organic eggs • Wild game 1 serving per week • Eggs	Avoid VIP plus: All eggs
Dairy	Dairy substitutes: almond, cashew, coconut, hazelnut, hemp, and rice milks with no sugar added	Cow's milk, cow's cheese, cheese with colorings, nondairy creamer, fruit yogurt, ice cream VIP "cheat": • Goat's milk/cheese • Sheep's milk/cheese • Unsweetened organic soy milk • Organic half & half or creamer • Kefir • Plain yogurt	Avoid VIP plus: All sheep milk/cheese All goat milk/cheese All soy milk/cheese All creamers All yogurts (Greek and kefir included)
Rice, Grains, Pasta	Amaranth; millet; buckwheat; quinoa; gluten-free pastas, tortillas, and wraps; rice crackers and cakes; amaranth breads; rice- or oat-based cereals; brown, white, red, or black rice	Gluten grains (barley, Kamut, rye, spelt, wheat), corn, oats, farro, semolina pasta VIP "cheat": • udon noodles • soba noodles • sprouted grain breads, flatbreads, pastas, and tortillas	Avoid VIP plus: All udon and soba noodles Sprouted grains and sprouted grain breads, flatbreads, pastas, and tortillas White rice—while it's great for healing GALT, it's high-glycemic so remove from diet if your goal is weight loss
Legumes (phytoestrogens, the most cancer-protective food we can eat! 1 to 3 servings a day)	All dried beans, peas, lentils, organic soy bean products like soy milk, tempe, soy nuts, tofu	Wasabi peas, protein powders with added sugars, canned beans with sugar or preservatives, bean dips with additives, non-organic soy, soy protein isolates VIP "cheat": Hummus and bean dips (read labels to ensure no added sugars, preservatives, or unhealthy oils)	Avoid VIP plus: All soy-based foods, which are common allergens
Vegetables (unlimited servings daily)	Nearly all fresh, frozen, or freshly juiced vegetables (not fried); greens recommended to clean out cells, seaweed, parsley, cilantro, garlic, onion, beets, artichokes, portobello and shiitake mushrooms	Corn, white potatoes, white mushrooms VIP "cheat": • Nightshades—tomatoes, peppers, potatoes, eggplant	Avoid VIP plus: All nightshades—tomatoes, peppers, potatoes, eggplant

Fruit (1 to 3 servings daily)	Fresh or frozen, dark-skinned fruits like red, blue, or purple berries, unsweetened apples, pears, peaches	Bottled fruit juice and drinks, fruit jams or spreads VIP "cheat": • Tomatoes • Citrus • Bananas	Avoid VIP plus: All citrus All tomatoes Bananas
Beverages (64 to 80 ounces minimum daily)	Spring and mineral waters in glass bottles, seltzer, herbal tea, yerba maté, green tea, ginseng tea, roasted grain coffee substitutes like chicory	Alcohol, soda and soft drinks, sports drinks, vitamin waters, coffee, caffeinated teas, fruit juice VIP "cheat": • Tap water • Distilled water • Coffee or tea (1–2 cups) • Fruit juice diluted 1:2	Avoid VIP plus: All coffee Tap or distilled water
Raw Nuts/Seeds (eaten sparingly as snacks)	Sunflower, sesame, and pumpkin seeds, sprouted seeds like alfalfa, radish, and sunflower, almonds, hazelnuts, pecans, walnuts, Brazil nuts, and their all-natural butters	Peanuts, peanut butter VIP "cheat": • Lightly roasted nuts and seeds • Pistachios	Avoid VIP plus: All roasted nuts/seeds Pistachios
Sweeteners	Stevia, Xylitol	Refined sugars, molasses, artificial sweeteners, cane juice powder, barley malt, amazake, rice syrup, fruit syrup VIP "cheat": • Agave nectar • Local honey • Natural fruit sugars	Avoid VIP plus: All honey Agave nectar
Spices and Condiments	Fermented products like fresh kimchi, fresh or dried herbs, and spices like garlic, pepper, and ginger, sea salt	Prepackaged seasonings, bottled ketchup, mustard, mayonnaise, olives, pickles, relish, salad dressings, capers, jarred sauces, malt vinegar, table salt VIP "cheat": • Non-malt vinegars like apple cider, balsamic	Avoid VIP plus: All vinegars
Fats and Oils (2 tbsp per day)	Olive oil and coconut oil only for cooking, flaxseed oil	Margarine, shortenings, spreads, peanut oil, vegetable oil, canola oil, olestra, clarified organic butter (ghee), all hydrogenated and partially hydrogenated fats and oils VIP "cheat": • cold-pressed oils • sesame oil • walnut oil • almond oil • safflower oil • pumpkin oil • avocado oil • organic butter	Avoid VIP plus: Butter

blood. (This is not a purging cleanse!) Proteins to avoid are casein and soy isolates because they're synthetic, irradiated, and genetically modified. Also avoid brands with added sugars, soy isolates, and casein or cow's milk proteins.

2. Gastrointestinal Repair Formula

These powerful combinations of herbs, amino acids, and enzymes act like a supercharger to your immunity and work to rebuild a strong gastrointestinal and immune lining (GALT) by regenerating its layers so more nutrients and fewer toxins and allergens are absorbed. The supported GALT provides a place for the probiotics to adhere to.

3. Probiotic Powder

A high-quality probiotic supplement provides *Lactobacillus acidophilus*, a good bacterium that lines the gut membranes and GALT. It helps digestion, absorption, and elimination of toxins and supports healthy immune function. The powder seals in GALT layers regenerated by the intestinal repair powder.

No probiotic powder? No problem. You can also get this healthy bacteria by eating fermented foods like sauerkraut, yogurt, kefir, and kimchi.

4. Green Food Powder or Green Juice

Concentrated green food supplements typically contain sea greens, green foods, fruits, and vegetables. Chlorophyll, the substance that makes plants green, acts like a chelating agent in our cells. This means it goes inside of our cells like a super sleuth and draws out toxins and heavy metals. Think of it like a cellular cleanser that, when finished, leaves you with a stronger immune system and far greater energy.

5. Fiber
A gentle soluble formula scrapes away the residue that accumulates on intestinal walls without inhibiting mineral absorption like many other insoluble fiber products such as psyllium do.

6. Organic Flaxseed Oil
Flaxseed oil is a vegetarian source of high-quality omega-3 fatty acids. The benefits of the omega-3 fatty acids include: inflammation support, hormone balance, fat-soluble vitamin support, healthy skin and hair, and cellular communication.

RxSTAR DETOX SHAKE

2 scoops Functional food powder (1 serving equ.)

2 teaspoons intestinal repair formula (or follow instructions on the bottle)

1 scoop green food powder (or follow instructions on the bottle) or

1 cup fresh-pressed green juice

½ teaspoon probiotic powder (or follow instructions on the bottle)

1 scoop fiber powder (or follow instructions on the bottle)

1 tablespoon flaxseed oil

¼ cup yogurt, rice milk, or almond milk (optional)

¼ cup frozen organic berries or fruit (optional)

Mix the above ingredients into 12 to 16 ounces of purified water. You may also add ice and blend. Take at least 30 to 60 minutes to drink this. It's a meal, don't chug it!

"When we were on the road with Neil Young a few years ago, there was a juicer in catering every day with a pile of fresh organic fruits and vegetables available for anyone to make juices. This was a revelation! A big fresh juice became a daily event and it was fantastic, and the way it made me feel led me to make it a regular part of my life. I bought a juicer as soon as I got home."

—PAT SANSONE, GUITARIST AND KEYBOARDS,
WILCO, AUTUMN DEFENSE

3 ADDITIONAL RxSTAR DETOX SUPPLEMENTS

You may need or want additional herbs or supplements to support this program. Below are some of the most beneficial supplements to consider:

1. Digestive Enzymes

Digestive enzymes support the function and production of our body's natural enzyme processes. In nonmedical lingo, that means they break down foods into smaller and more absorbable nutrients, so you get more bang for your bite.

Digestive Enzymes: Take 1 tablet at lunch and dinner. Look for vegetarian enzyme formulas that support the digestion of fats, carbohydrates, and proteins in the pancreas and small intestine.

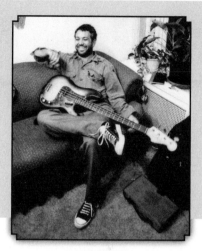

MIKE WATT
(DANNY CLINCH)

2. Laxative/Bowel Stimulants

Gentle herbal laxatives may be necessary if you find that you are not eliminating through the bowels daily. We're talking once after each meal. Otherwise, toxins released from your cells and organs stay in your colon.

- **SEVERAL HERBAL BRANDS WORK BRILLIANTLY.** Choose one that strengthens the wall of the intestines, so you can eliminate regularly.
- **MAGNESIUM CITRATE ALSO WORKS.** Start with 500 mg before bed.

"You need fucking fiber, you know! I drink that orange-tasting thing! There's a real deficiency in the regular chow, you know? It comes up on you getting older. You know all of this is the husk of some seed on the grass. It keeps you regular, it keeps you happy!"

—MIKE WATT, BASSIST,

THE MINUTEMEN, FIREHOSE, IGGY POP AND THE STOOGES

3. Electrolyte Replacement

Electrolytes support the proper mineral balance in the body and promote excellent hydration. It's a good idea to take an electrolyte formula daily during the detox especially if you're doing the recommended saunas, steams, colonics, and exercises that promote water loss.

> Emergen-C: 1 to 2 packets per day mixed with water.
> Coconut water with no sugars added. Fresh coconuts are ideal.

HARM REDUCTION TECHNIQUE: ELECTRO-LIGHTS

Electrolyte replacement drinks can be a great way to restore lost minerals, but many popular sports drinks like Gatorade are sugar and chemical bombs. Emergen-C is my favorite electrolyte powder and is much lower in sugar. Other natural sources of electrolytes are coconut water, soup broths, bouillon, and miso soup. Sure, you won't pound these while you're on the treadmill, but they're perfect for staying hydrated after you hit the gym.

HERBS, SPICES, AND ESSENTIAL OILS TO SUPPORT DETOXIFICATION

Detoxification is a natural healing process so it only makes sense that Mother Nature provides herbs and spices that can support your system. Toss them into your shakes. Blend and make them into herbal teas that can be drunk hot or cold. Or take herbs as supplements in tincture or capsule forms. Another option is to add their essential oils to your massage lotions for additional detox support.

Different herbs support different organ systems in removing toxins. Here's a quick breakdown of which herbs aid specific functions:

LUNGS: lungwort, lobelia, chlorella, elecampane, mullein

LYMPHATIC SYSTEM: red clover, cleavers, gallium, astragalus, prickly ash, licorice root

KIDNEYS AND URINARY TRACT: gravel root, uva ursi, juniper berries, burdock root, parsley, nettles

BLOOD AND SKIN: burdock root, yellow dock, Oregon grape root, sarsaparilla, stinging nettles

GASTROINTESTINAL TRACT: marshmallow root, turkey rhubarb, gentian, cascara sagrada, ginger, dandelion root, licorice root, garlic

LIVER AND GALLBLADDER: milk thistle, artichoke, dandelion, red clover, turmeric, basil, rosemary, juniper

Add these additional delicious herbs and spices to meals, teas, shakes, and sauces to kick up flavor and support your cleanse:

Cardamom

Cayenne

Cilantro

Cinnamon

Onion

Oregano

Parsley

Thyme

"I always try to eat organic, well-sourced meats, fish, and vegetables, and combine foods for maximum nutrition whether touring or at home. That said, I also eat for flavor and pleasure, balancing fresh and seasonal veggies, salads, grains, starches, and meats. I recommend a very exciting vegetarian cookbook, *Plenty* by Yotam Ottolenghi, for healthy, tasty home cooking."

—JORDAN McLEAN, TRUMPETER, FIRE OF SPACE

GIVE CREDENCE TO THE CLEARWATER REVIVAL

Water is the most abundant nutrient in the body, comprising at least two-thirds of our mass, yet it is one of the biggest nutritional deficiencies in the average diet. It's quite the paradox. If most of us knew that it is a primary component in every bodily function and carries our electrolytes, we might be more diligent about getting our minimum sixty-four ounces every day.

But not all H_2O is created equal! Check out all of the contaminants you may be drinking from an unfiltered tap:

Aluminum

Antibiotics

Asbestos

Bacteria

Cadmium

Chlorine

Fluoride

Industrial chemicals

Lead

Medications

Mercury

Nitrates

Organic solvents

Parasites

Pesticides

Radon

Sodium

Viruses

Arm yourself against these toxins by drinking water purified by carbon block filters, which leave minerals intact, so you get spring-water-like benefits without the microorganisms.

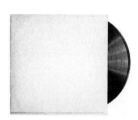

BONUS TRACKS

"As a roots man, I tend to eat the basics at a conscious and moderate pace, sort of a no-gimmick diet, conscious and logical."

—DARRYL JENIFER, BASSIST, **BAD BRAINS**

"From time to time I fast with a modified version on the Master Cleanse. I add green vegetable smoothies as well as vegetable protein drinks made with coconut water, hemp powder, açai powder, and noni powder."

—DARRYL JONES, BASSIST, **THE ROLLING STONES**

"Let me tell you something. . . . I go to the doctor for my checkups and blood pressure. But I don't like how they tell you to take this pill and take that pill. You start taking one pill and then soon you are taking ten! If you know what I mean! I bought myself a juicer so I can get some vitamins for my body and clean things out. You know what I'm sayin'?"

—SHARON JONES, SINGER,

SHARON JONES & THE DAP-KINGS

"I like to think, 'Reduce, reuse. Recycle as a last resort.' I have a reusable one-quart juice glass that I keep filled with water. There are so many wasted water bottles on tour. If you collected every half-drunk water bottle on a tour I bet you could quench the dying thirst of a small country. I wish we could change that."

—SAMEER BHATTACHARYA, SINGER, SONGWRITER, FLYLEAF

CHAPTER 6

DETOX YOUR BODY, MIND, AND HOME

"The power of the mind is incredible. Keeping yourself positive and being kind to other people is priceless! What I think will change the world ultimately is the inner revolution."

JESSY GREENE, VIOLINIST, PINK, THE FOO FIGHTERS

C hanges you make to your body on the inside need to be supported by your outside environment. If you detox your diet but not your mind, body, and home, you won't get the full benefit of the cleanse. As we discussed in chapter 1, your mind and body are interconnected. What you eat is just as important as how you live, what you think, and who is in your life. Over the next three weeks, just as you are detoxing from the inside out, you will also examine the ways in which these three areas can be examined and decluttered. The cleaner the slate you create, the stronger the foundation for building optimal health in all areas of your life.

PHASE 1: DETOX YOUR BODY

Specific exercises and body treatments will aid the detox process. Not only do they help move out the physical toxins; they also help to purge emotional toxins like stress and anxiety. Some of these exercises and activities you may already do, and others, like massage, you're probably just waiting for an "official" excuse to add to your life!

DETOX YOUR BODY CHECKLIST

✔ Aerobics: 15 minutes, 3–7 days per week
✔ Body scrubs: 1 time per month
✔ Castor oil pack: 30 minutes, 1 time per month
✔ Colon hydrotherapy: 1 session per month
✔ Epsom salt baths: 20 minutes, 1 time per week
✔ Hot/cold shower or baths: 10 minutes hot, 3 minutes cold. Repeat.
✔ Massage therapy: 1 session per week or month
✔ Skin brushing: 1 minute daily in shower
✔ Steam or sauna: 10–20 minutes, 2 days per week
✔ Walking: 20 minutes daily
✔ Yoga and stretching: 15 minutes daily

> "I remember waking up and looking in the mirror and going, who is that? This does not look like me. I don't know who those puffy eyes are. This is not me! That is when I meditate, do yoga, and hang upside down because any inversion pose can really help with your puffiness."
> —JESSY GREENE, VIOLINIST, PINK, THE FOO FIGHTERS

RxSTAR REMEDY DETOX EXERCISE

Regular exercise and movement is essential during your detox. The recommendations below promote circulation of the blood and lymph, which enhances the cleansing of the blood and immune system. Toxins from the muscles, skin, and organs can be moved into the blood, where they are then eliminated from the body through the support of the liver, gut, and urinary tract.

During your detox, movement should be gentle and focused on releasing stress and tension. There should be minimal concentration on strength training. Consistency will yield the best results, so try to do something every day. And because the core of this program is YOU, be sure to do workouts you enjoy!

Aerobic Exercise

20 minutes, 3 days per week

Aerobic exercise gets your heart rate up, improves your circulation, and strengthens your immune system by circulating the lymphatic fluid. It's also the fastest natural high you can get: aerobic exercise promotes the release of endorphins, which are natural painkillers and feel-good molecules. During the detox, focus on mild activities, like swimming, jogging, dancing, biking, or hiking. Don't push yourself if you're feeling weak, and, again, do what you enjoy.

"Swimming laps is a full-body workout, and it also has a meditative quality that is good for me while on the road. Just having at least an hour a day of being quiet, in the moment, and away from cell phones, computers, and the noise and intensity of the tour is invaluable."

—PAT SANSONE, GUITARIST AND KEYBOARDS,

WILCO, AUTUMN DEFENSE

HARM REDUCTION TECHNIQUE: BEND A LITTLE

Stretch when you're already warmed up. There's been a lot of controversy brewing about the benefits of stretching before and after exercise. In my practice, I've seen great benefits in the flexibility, performance, injury reduction, and overall health of my clients by adding this practice. The key is to stretch when muscles are warm to prevent strain, muscle tears, or overflexion. Start by doing leg lifts, gentle side stretches, even walking. Just five minutes increases circulation enough to prep your body for deeper stretching.

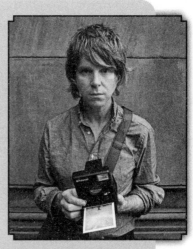

PAT SANSONE
(DANNY CLINCH)

THE ROCKSTAR REMEDY

Walking

15–20 minutes daily

When walking, swing your arms with the opposite leg (that is, your right arm with your left leg, and vice versa). There's a method to the madness: emphasizing opposite sides of the body at the same time coordinates the left and right brain hemispheres and engages our upper body to pump and drain the lymphatics.

Yoga and Stretching

10–15 minutes daily

Most forms of vigorous exercise stimulate the systems of detoxification. But yoga, with its focus on systematically stretching and compressing every part of the body, naturally keeps waste-removal departments of the body functioning well. You could say that many of the poses really do squeeze out the toxins.

Yoga aids in mental detox as well. Emotions like stress, fear, anxiety, and depression are carried in the cells and tissues of your body. Yoga clears toxic and stagnant thoughts by releasing stress and supports the elimination of mental chatter so that your mind may be free from stressful thinking.

"My main health regimen is yoga. It is mostly about meditation and the spiritual for me. I do my stretching poses every day as a prelude to meditation and the health benefits are extraordinary. I try and meditate for a couple hours daily. It's not always possible to do that much, but I nearly always get in a good amount."

—JEFF PILSON, BASSIST, FOREIGNER

RxSTAR REMEDY DETOX TREATMENTS AND BODYWORK

Work done externally can take internal cleansing to a deeper level and add some interesting and exhilarating new habits to your healthy lifestyle. Try them at least once during the program.

Body Scrubs and Exfoliations

Once per month

This is your ticket to radiance. Fibrous materials or natural salt or sugar-based mixes exfoliate and clear dead cells on the skin's surface to allow regeneration of underlying layers. You'll improve the youthfulness and elasticity of your skin, making it look younger, healthier, and brighter.

Castor Oil Packs

30 minutes, once per week

Castor oil—that sticky oil extracted from the castor bean—has a long tradition in natural medicine as support for cleansing the liver, gallbladder, lymph, and large intestines. Used topically, it softens and breaks down scar tissue and adhesions. To use, massage a quarter-size dab into your lower abdomen below the ribs. Next, cover with a towel-wrapped hot water bottle or heating pad for 30–40 minutes to improve absorption into your body.

Colon Hydrotherapy

1 session per week or month

Colon irrigation cleanses the large intestine with purified water in order to remove residual toxins and wastes that accumulate on the walls of the intestines and cause constipation and toxicity. If you're uncomfortable with such an "intimate" treatment, don't worry, it's not a necessity for a successful detox. Just know that if you do try it, you'll feel much lighter and clearer afterward.

Epsom Salt or Sea Salt Baths

20 minutes, 1 time per week

Epsom and sea salts are both luxurious and healthy. High in magnesium and other minerals, they relax muscles and calm the mind, while removing toxins like lactic acid from soft tissues. That soreness and fatigue you feel after a day on your feet or at the gym? It will disappear after a soak in these healing salts. Their best-kept secret, however, is their ability to remove and neutralize radiation from computers, cell phones, televisions, and more. Soak 20 minutes in warm water mixed with 2 cups of salts. Relax and visualize stress leaving your body.

Massage Therapy

1 session per week or month

There's a reason that there are massage tables backstage at nearly all festivals and concerts—and no, it's not because rock stars are divas. Massage is one of the best things you can do for your mind and body, particularly during detox. The treatment improves the circulation and detoxification of the cells, blood, and lymphatics. It also releases stored tension that accumulates in your muscles, which you experience as painful spasms and knots.

Skin Brushing

1 minute daily

Lightly stroke wet or dry skin in the direction of the heart using a loofah or netlike sponge. Doing so promotes detoxification and circulation of the lymphatics and strengthens immunity. Remember to use a light hand—you're increasing lymphatic flow, not removing dead skin layers.

Steam or Sauna

10–20 minutes, 2 days per week

Okay, I probably don't have to convince you to add a little spa time to your weekly routine. A lot of gyms these days have saunas or steam rooms. If not, turn on the hot water in your shower and close your bathroom door . . . get it as steamy as you can take. These treatments cause you to sweat, which removes toxins that have accumulated in your fat cells, skin, and blood. Deep sweating, in fact, is the best way to eliminate pesticides, plastics, and heavy metals from your body.

If you have high or low blood pressure or other medical conditions, consult your physician before using the steam or sauna. For those in good health, use the steam or sauna for 10–20 minutes at a time and have an electrolyte drink (raw coconut water or Emergen-C) to prevent dehydration.

PHASE 2: DETOX YOUR MIND

"I chant twice a day—that is critical to me. I started chanting more than twenty years ago, but I never chanted twice a day. I see the results in my life from chanting twice a day and making that practice consistent. It completely changed my life in so my ways. Little ways and big ways."

—COURTNEY LOVE, SINGER, SONGWRITER, MUSICIAN

No matter what type of changes you make in your life, it's important to make sure they stick by getting your brain on board, too. Your mind plays a huge role in your ability to heal and to reach your health goals.

Cleansing your mind, emotions, and spirit of things that are no longer useful to you will accelerate healing throughout your body. When you release negative relationships, emotions, and thoughts, you create space for a newer energy and experience that aligns with your elevated state of health. You'll see that your body is an important vessel for transformation of the mind and spirit, too.

When we are plagued by anxiety from negative thinking, we tend to hold our breath or breathe shallow breaths. This causes an accumulation of carbon dioxide in our cells, which creates a buildup of acidity. Releasing negativity and worry can improve our breath and increase the circulation of oxygen in our bodies and brains. Life-giving oxygen makes the future look brighter and clearer.

The practices below can help you release thoughts and patterns that aren't pushing you toward the positive spectrum of health. Choose whichever ones resonate with your belief systems and lifestyle.

Meditation

Meditation allows you to quiet and focus your mind. It releases the extraneous thoughts that constantly bombard your psyche and cause undue tension and stress. The practice is sort of like a cleansing bath that lets you enjoy the present moment to its fullest. It's one of the most popular methods musicians use to prepare themselves for a performance. Meditation styles vary and may or may not be associated with a spiritual tradition. There are many books, apps, audio guides, and classes available for a beginner. Look for a variation that suits your beliefs and lifestyle.

Mindfulness

Mindfulness is the art of complete awareness and attention to the present moment. Much of our attention is spent reliving our past and worrying about the future. When we do this we cannot truly benefit from the gift of the present moment. Mindfulness can be practiced by anyone and it is not a religion.

I am a big fan of the Vietnamese Buddhist monk Thich Nhat Hanh. He has many wonderful books that help bring the practice of mindfulness to every activity of our daily lives. One great book is called *Peace Is Every Step*—it's perfect for beginners who want to learn how mindfulness can be integrated into their lives.

"I have my own spiritual ideas and they work for me. I feel that the human mind is probably unable to comprehend what's actually taking place on the spiritual plane in its entirety. That belief system has always taken care of me when I've put my faith in it. But I've never tried to figure it out. Whatever "it" is. I loved Eckhart Tolle's Power of Now. People like us have a very hard time staying in the Now. Just being conscious of the fact that you're not in the moment can bring you back to it."

—DAVE NAVARRO, GUITARIST, JANE'S ADDICTION

HARM REDUCTION TECHNIQUE: TO BE OR NOT TO BE

Instead of thinking of where else you could be when you travel or commute, stay in the moment. Meditate, listen to music, catch up on reading, send emails, or make calls. You're being given the gift of personal time, so use it to your advantage rather than worrying about when you're going to get "there."

Personal Inventory

Take a personal inventory of the thoughts, emotions, and behaviors that may no longer be useful to you or that may be holding you back. This awareness is the first step. Be open to ideas of how destructive patterns may be eliminated or transformed. Let go of resentments. Spending too much time focusing on the past prevents you from redirecting your energy to create a healthy, vibrant present and future.

Now is also the time to release negative or self-destructive thought patterns or self-criticism. For example, "I can't" becomes "I can." Follow with a new positive intention. Soon the "I can't" gets completely replaced with a powerful declaration. You are your own best advocate.

Prayer

Prayer, a form of connecting to our higher power or God, is practiced in all religions. It's a way of releasing your burdens, concerns, and worries by giving them over to a power or consciousness greater than you. Because the practice can help you feel safe, protected, and cared for, it can be a great tool during detox for releasing fear, stress, or anxiety. Prayer focused on forgiveness is essential during the detox period. Forgiveness of others and of self is equally important.

Psychotherapy

If you're seeing a therapist, see if you can focus a few of your sessions during the detox on releasing toxic behaviors and emotions. If you're not in therapy but need guidance in processing unresolved issues, the detox is a perfect time to start. Guided support can be invaluable in transforming your past and relieving old wounds.

Goodbye Negativity, Hello Happiness

Certainly there are many ways to cultivate bliss. Some take days, others can take a lifetime. Below is a quick, easy, and almost painless checklist of happiness boosters, designed to free your mind, unleash joy, and release habits or feelings holding you back. Try them for added oomph during the detox:

- **ABSTAIN FROM ADDICTIONS.** Yes, TV, Internet, and shopping are included. Basically anything you do for four or more hours that distracts you from *living* can be unhealthy.
- **AVOID DRAINING RELATIONSHIPS.** Just say "no" to the person, invite, or obligation that makes you anxious just thinking about it. And don't feel bad about it. Life is too short to be filled with things and people we dread.
- **ELIMINATE SELF-LOATHING AND SELF-CRITICISM.** You are taking a huge step to do something positive for yourself— you should feel great about that.
- **PROCESS GRIEF AND LOSS.** If you haven't taken the time to heal from a major trauma, now is the time to acknowledge the pain you've been carrying around, and find ways to let it go.

Relationships

Detox is the time to have a heart-to-heart with yourself. Which relationships don't support who you are and the lifestyle you want to lead? It may be the time to move your attention away from the ones that aren't working for you or are draining you. It also may be time to forgive (starting with yourself), clear the air with loved ones, and let go of resentments eating away at you. Look closely at the people in your life, from coworkers to family to friends. How can you transform any negative situations into something more positive for everyone?

My favorite quote from the U2 song "Walk On" is "Love is an easy thing, the only baggage that you bring . . . is all that you can't leave behind." I love this because it allows us to reflect on what judgments and perceptions from our past we bring into relationships. We all have had hardships and challenges but they are only "baggage" if we are bringing them into our current relationships. Consider your part in your relationships and what you may be bringing from the past that needs to be left behind so that you can cultivate a healthy relationship in the present.

Sleep

Most people live in a semi-constant state of sleep deprivation. When you operate on 10 percent, you function at 10 percent. That's not how rock stars, or you, are able to perform at their peak. When they're on tour, my busiest clients sneak in catnaps whenever and wherever they can. When we sleep, our bodies go into a deep state of renewal and rejuvenation. When cleansing, most of the liver's detoxification happens at night when we're out cold but our body is working overtime.

"I know myself and I know I'm not likely to get eight hours of sleep at night so I try to supplement that during the day by taking naps or just shutting down for a couple hours. I don't have the luxury any more of getting high. Through some strange turn of events, naptime has become an opiate. It's become my way to shut my brain off. I'm not a religious guy but there is no finer cure for insomnia than reading the Bible. Why do you think there's a copy in every hotel in the world? Crack that open and you'll be out in a flash."
—DAVE NAVARRO, GUITARIST, JANE'S ADDICTION

Over the next 21 days, get a minimum of 8–10 hours of sleep per night, and if you can, shoot for 10–12 hours for deeper healing. That may sound like a pipe dream, but it's only three weeks. Don't feel guilty if you need more rest during the detox period—that's normal initially because your body requires so much extra energy to eliminate toxins. Even if you're the creative, nocturnal type, it is best to fall asleep before midnight and sleep while it's dark for normal hormone and neurotransmitter balance. This will help with your stress hormones as well. Turn off the TV or computer an hour or two earlier and enjoy some extra z's.

Spiritual Detox

Most religions and spiritual practices incorporate some form of cleansing and detoxification into the traditions. If you have such a ritual, you may want to incorporate that into your detox, which can enhance traditions that are already part of your life. Some examples include fasting, confession, taking inventory, baptism, and forgiveness.

PHASE 3: DETOX YOUR LIFE

Most of us have no idea how many harmful substances we are exposed to in our homes and in the products we use. From furniture to soaps and cleaners to cosmetics, it's truly mind-boggling how many chemicals we encounter each day. The good news is that the majority of these environmental toxins can be easily eliminated, and removing them will do wonders for your physical, mental, and emotional health. The transition to natural products may cause sticker shock at first, because you will probably need to purchase items you don't currently have, but the investment in your health will be worth it: The less exposure you have to toxic chemicals and habits, the fewer medical bills you should have.

DETOX-YOUR-LIFE CHECKLIST

✔ Deep-clean the house from the top to the bottom, saving the floor and carpet for last.

- ✔ Get 20–30 minutes of sunlight per day.
- ✔ Open windows to exchange stale air with fresh.
- ✔ Remove and recycle clutter from all rooms in your house.
- ✔ Remove toxic cleaning products.
- ✔ Remove toxic personal care products.
- ✔ Sleep 8–10 hours per night.
- ✔ Start a "no shoes indoors" policy to keep dirt and debris outside.
- ✔ Set up a recycling system in your house and yard.
- ✔ Use biodegradable cellulose sponges available in natural stores.
- ✔ Use headsets with cell phones.
- ✔ Use radiation guards on computers.

HARM REDUCTION TECHNIQUE: SNEAK IN YOUR Z'S

Studies show that 30-minute disco naps can help you make up for lost sleep. It's one of the secret weapons of rock stars on tour. I also recommend what I call "lost sleep sessions" for the seriously snooze-deprived. If I've pulled several straight days with little sleep, I'll give myself one day to crash for several hours straight. It's a great way to rejuvenate when you can squeeze in a day off.

Unplugged: Detox Your Technology

Some of the greatest health risks we're exposed to aren't the ones we can see and touch. Radiation exposure is a real risk with the electronics we use each day, such as your computer, smartphone, and television. Fortunately, there are some basic things you can do to protect yourself.

Use a headset or Bluetooth when talking on a cell phone and position the device one to two feet away from your body. This reduces microwave radiation by about 80 percent. Also, turn off your data plan unless using the Internet; otherwise you're constantly drawing unnecessary radiation. Text instead of talk when possible; it is less harmful.

Be sure to have a radiation guard on your computer screen. Desktops are healthier than laptops, which give off a more concentrated amount of radiation and are often placed directly on our laps. During the detox, avoid unnecessary Internet surfing and take a walk with a friend instead.

Speaking of limiting screen time, turning off the TV during the detox limits radiation exposure and gives you more space for socializing. Trust me, your favorite shows will still be available 21 days from now.

Last but not least: Start replacing free-radical-emitting fluorescent lightbulbs in your home with full-spectrum bulbs, which imitate sunlight. You'll boost your mood and immune system at the same time.

"Creativity is always with you. Creativity is really based around what you find interesting, what fascinates you and then describing what you think or feel about that using artistic interpretation. The discipline is in learning how to shift one's focus towards that which is interesting for an extended period of time without allowing distraction. Soft addictions such as television, Facebook, and the telephone are devastating distractions to creativity. Not that these things shouldn't be enjoyed, but there is a time and place for everything."
—GEOFF TATE, SINGER, QUEENSRŸCHE

Housecleaning: Detox Your Space

Cleaning doesn't have to be a dirty word. In fact, if you use this time to deep-clean and clear clutter, you'll free up not just physical space, but mental and emotional space, too. First on the hit list? Recycling or donating all the clothes, appliances, and other items that you do not use anymore. Next, filing away the clutter: CDs, books, papers, anything creating mental chaos. Third, replace chemical-laden cleaning products with brands that are nontoxic, environmentally safe, natural, and effective. Finally, clear your home of xeno-estrogens, toxic substances found in the environment that mimic estrogen in your body and can cause cancer. I call them the 3 P's, and they should always be avoided:

1. Pesticides (in foods)
2. Petroleum in products we put on our skin
3. Plastic bottles for water and other beverages.

HARM REDUCTION TECHNIQUE: CLEAN UP YOUR KITCHEN

Never cook or bake with aluminum. It is a common toxin that is associated with cancer and Alzheimer's disease. Instead, use stainless steel, glass, or ceramic pots or pans.

HARM REDUCTION TECHNIQUE: SWAP YOUR TOOTHPASTE

Switch to a natural, fluoride-free brand of toothpaste. Fluoride is a neurotoxin that interferes with your thyroid gland's ability to bind with iodine, which is necessary to produce thyroid hormone.

Once you've detoxed your space, find products with no secrets, ones that provide a complete list of ingredients. You want them to be:

- BIODEGRADABLE
- CERTIFIED BY AN INDEPENDENT THIRD PARTY: ECOLOGO (ENVIRONMENTALCHOICE.COM) OR GREEN SEAL (GREENSEAL.ORG)
- CONCENTRATED, TO REDUCE PACKAGING MATERIALS
- FREE OF ADDED DYES (EXCEPT WHEN ADDED FOR SAFETY PURPOSES)
- FREE OF SKIN IRRITANTS
- FREE OF VOCs (VOLATILE ORGANIC COMPOUNDS)
- MADE FROM NATURAL CLEANERS, SUCH AS CITRUS, SEED, VEGETABLE, AND PINE OILS
- NITROGEN-FREE
- NON-TOXIC
- PERFUME- AND FRAGRANCE-FREE
- PHOSPHATE-FREE
- VEGETABLE-BASED SURFACTANTS

Essential Oils: Spice Up Your Surroundings

Essential oils are derived from plants—they're the oils that give any plant or flower its wonderful smell. Not only do essential oils smell incredible, but they also offer fantastic health benefits. Put a few drops of an essential oil into your bath or body moisturizer, or add them to oil diffusers to freshen your home or office.

When it comes to detox support, these antioxidant-rich oils are rock stars:

- BASIL
- CEDAR

- JUNIPER
- LEMON
- OREGANO
- PEPPERMINT
- ROSEMARY
- SAGE
- THYME

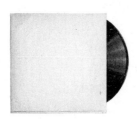

BONUS TRACKS

SULLY'S GINGER BATH BOMB

"This recipe is from back in my wilder days.

1. Drink 2 quarts of spring water
2. Fill up a bathtub with hot water
3. Add 1 cup of baking soda
4. Add 1 freshly cut ginger root
5. And 10 drops of essential oil of peppermint

Get in that baby and it will suck the toxins right out of your body. Be careful you don't pass out! You may even need a spotter!"

—BILL SULLIVAN, TOUR MANAGER

CHARLEY DRAYTON'S GINGER/GARLIC POULTICE

"This can be used on any place that you have pain or injury. You put it on the open part of your body and it sucks the toxins out.

1. Get some fresh ginger, garlic, and onion
2. Chop them up
3. Wrap the mixture in a thin cloth
4. Steep it in hot water
5. Wrap it in Saran Wrap
6. Lay it on the part of your body that is sore.

Don't worry, your friends will still love you if they know you are trying to take care of yourself!"

—CHARLEY DRAYTON, DRUMMER, BASSIST, AND PRODUCER,
FIONA APPLE, NEIL YOUNG, KEITH RICHARDS

"Anytime I'm creatively low or blocked, I take my dogs for a run in our canyon in Santa Monica. There's something magical about running on a trail in the wilderness that allows the creative to flow for me. Its very cleansing."

—RAINE MAIDA, SINGER, SONGWRITER, OUR LADY PEACE

"I did acupuncture and massage during chemo [for breast cancer], which helped a lot with the side effects. I now get monthly massages. Playing my accordion is very hard on my back and shoulders especially since I am taking a medication [for cancer prevention] that creates muscle soreness and arthritis symptoms."

—JENNY CONLEE, ACCORDIONIST, DECEMBERISTS

"The important thing is just really enjoying the present moment. It starts with the breath. You don't have to think about any temples or any golden statues, or have to wrap yourself in a particular kind of clothing, or have that perfect pillow and the perfect music. You're supposed to just meditate with the goal of connecting with the oneness of the universe. And not be thinking, Okay, I'm going to be a Buddhist or a Hindu right now. People get hung up on the accouterments, but it really just comes down to connecting."

—GARY LOURIS, SINGER, SONGWRITER, GUITARIST, THE JAYHAWKS

"The two things that helped me kick anxiety were, first, learning how to say no. And, second, giving up alcohol. Because for years, I thought that drinking was the cure for my anxiety, which of course was a lie. Since I quit drinking, I've learned how to relax more. . . . I used to be a micromanager in the studio. Now I just stand out of the way and let talented musicians do their thing. I just need to play the guitar. And trust."

—ERNIE CUNNINGHAM, AKA "ERNIE C," BODY COUNT

"We do our best with environmental friendliness, although on tour, a lot is simply beyond our control. We can all affect the environment by doing simple things like turning off lights and TVs, not letting the faucet run, reusing and recycling. When everyone does their part, a lot of great green things happen."

—KEVIN CRONIN, SINGER, GUITARIST, REO SPEEDWAGON

"I do get massages and regularly use essential oils like peppermint. I relax myself by lying down and doing some visualization exercises that I learned in acting class. Exercising is the best thing. It gets my metabolism going and helps with depression and fatigue."

—RICKIE LEE JONES, SINGER, SONGWRITER

"A positive attitude has made a difference in my career, yes. Being grateful comes easy to me. My sense of gratitude comes from growing up with the Good Book. I grew up reading the Bible. Still do. I'm partial to Philippians 4:6–7. 'Do not be anxious about anything, but in every situation, by prayer and petition, with thanksgiving, present your requests to God.' Put all your burdens on God."

—FRED COURY, DRUMMER, CINDERELLA

"If you look closely onstage, you won't see water bottles, as we all drink from canteens. In conjunction with Reverb, an environmentally sustainable tour group, we mandate recyclable materials and invest in green grants to help smaller bands plan environmentally sustainable tours. We also participate in Reverb's Farm to Stage Program, where, whenever possible, all of our in-house food and catering is provided by local farms."

—BRANDI CARLILE, SINGER, SONGWRITER, PIANO, GUITARIST

"Depression is a terrible thing. I never had it until I lost my sons through a divorce battle. I take a lot of anger and frustration out on my guitar. My music makes me happy, my animals are wonderful, and I try to surround myself with good, happy, encouraging people with NO DRAMA! I do things that make me feel good, like shopping, hanging with close friends who make me laugh—laughter is a good antidepressant."

—LITA FORD, GUITARIST, THE RUNAWAYS

"In these times you have to be really aware of meat. If you're going to eat it, think of it like a drug. You better know who the dealer is. You better know who's dealing that meat."

—**LYDIA LUNCH**, SINGER, PERFORMER, AUTHOR, POET

PART THREE

NOURISH AND REVIVE

CHAPTER 7

STAGE TWO: HEALTH FOOD ROCKS!

N ow that you've finished the detox and have been on your best behavior, it's time to adapt your new healthy habits for the real world. Choosing whole, unprocessed, and organic foods—the "magic elixirs" of my plan—gives your body what it needs for optimal health, increased stamina, sharper focus, and overall vitality.

It's time to put the 90/10 Rule into practice. It's the only food guideline I ask you to follow. It will be your secret to staying energetic and healthy despite all the strains you put on your body by living a demanding lifestyle. The RxStar Remedy diet is this simple: 10 percent of the time you indulge in what you want. You don't worry or limit yourself when it comes to the foods you love. Yes, that includes a glass of wine at dinner or a chocolate croissant for breakfast. You savor and enjoy the good things in life. The other 90 percent of the time you're mindful about what you eat, following the food recommendations listed in this chapter and avoiding the junk that sabotages your health.

Put this one practice into place and I promise you that you'll feel so fantastic, you won't even want to ditch your healthy habits 10 percent of the time. If this sounds challenging, don't worry. There's a realistic and manageable way to ensure success: start immediately, start small. That's right. Find one or two simple changes you're confident you can make today and then set corresponding long-term goals that help you stay motivated to make larger transformations over time. I often ask my clients to pick one simple step first, such as switching out sugary drinks for more water. They feel so good after only a week that they're willing to make more short- and long-term changes.

RxSTAR FOOD QUIZ: DO YOU EAT LIKE A RxSTAR?

As we discussed, there are many paradigms around food. We have moved from seeing food as merely energy and calories to seeing food as nutrition, medicine, and information. The choices we make around food can determine whether the food we are eating is causing disease, giving us nutrition, or providing medicine that can aid our healing.

The following quiz will help you identify the places where your diet may be lacking. Is the food you eat promoting wellness or disease? Is it moving you closer toward the "healthy" end of the spectrum or pulling you toward the "disease" end?

I encourage you to take the quiz before you begin your RxStar Remedy changes. Then one to two months later you can retake it to see how the changes to your diet have influenced you. Hopefully, you will notice that you have learned to choose "Food as Medicine" for at least 90 percent of the time.

1. I drink water
   A. that is filtered with a carbon block purifier.

B. from the tap

C. in plastic bottles

2. The amount of water I drink is:
   A. 8–10 glasses per day
   B. 4–6 glasses per day
   C. fewer than 4 glasses per day

3. My primary beverages are:
   A. water and herbal teas
   B. juices and water
   C. soda and soft drinks

4. I eat fruits and vegetables:
   A. 5–7 servings per day
   B. 2–3 servings per day
   C. fewer than 2 servings per day

5. I eat fruits and vegetables that are:
   A. mostly organic
   B. not organic but I wash the skins
   C. not organic but are usually canned

6. I eat fruits and vegetables that are:
   A. a variety of colors daily
   B. the same colors every day
   C. so processed that I can't see the color

7. I eat nuts and seeds that are:
   A. organic, salt-free, and raw
   B. salted and raw
   C. salted and roasted

8. I eat beans and legumes that are:
   A. organic and home-cooked
   B. canned
   C. refried and packaged in spreads

9. I eat breads that are made with:
   A. organic, gluten-free, or sprouted grains
   B. whole wheat or whole grains
   C. white flour

10. I eat cereals that are made with:
    A. oats, quinoa, or rice
    B. whole-wheat flour
    C. white flour and sugars

11. The primary grains in my diet are:
    A. organic brown rice, quinoa, oats, and millet
    B. whole wheat, white rice, and oats
    C. white flour in breads and pastas and white rice

12. The primary dairy products that I consume are:
    A. organic cow's cheese and yogurt
    B. organic cow's milk
    C. non-organic cow's cheese, yogurt, and milk

13. I eat ice cream that is made with:
    A. coconut milk, goat milk, and rice milk
    B. organic cow's milk
    C. non-organic cow's milk

14. The choices of eggs I eat are:
    A. organic eggs only
    B. non-organic eggs
    C. Egg Beaters

15. I eat chicken and poultry that are:
    A. organic and free-range only
    B. non-organic
    C. packaged or processed, like lunch meats; or fried

16. I eat seafood and fish that are:
    A. wild and sustainable and low in mercury
    B. farmed primarily
    C. canned and deep fried

17. The red meat that I eat is:
    A. organic and grass fed
    B. non-organic
    C. processed (lunch meats and other processed meats)

18. I fry my foods with the following oils:
    A. organic butter, coconut oil, and olive oils
    B. olive oils and non-organic butter
    C. vegetable oils

19. I use salad dressings that are made with:
    A. organic olive, flax, or cold-pressed vegetable or nut oils
    B. olive oil
    C. vegetable oils and hydrogenated oils

20. The sweeteners that I use in food include:
   A. stevia, honey, agave nectar, and organic sweeteners
   B. refined sugars and brown sugars
   C. artificial sweeteners such as aspartame, Splenda, and saccharin

If you answered (a) to more than 15 questions then your food is primarily your medicine.

If you answered (a) and (b) to 10–15 questions then food is providing you with nutrition, but there is room for improvement.

If you answered (b) or (c) to more than 15 questions then your food choices may be promoting disease and disharmony in your body.

My goal for my clients—and you—is to help you understand how you got to where you are, what you can do to feel better, and how to keep your health optimized over time. Use your results of the quiz above as a starting point for success.

WHAT TO EAT: 16 FOODS THAT FUEL YOUR RxSTAR LIFESTYLE

There are no magic tricks or gimmicks. If you eat foods from the list below 90 percent of the time, you'll nourish and revive your mind, body, and spirit and feel your vitality soar.

> "I try not to eat any 'whites.' That would be refined sugars, wheat, white rice, dairy, etc. Fresh-pressed juices are my new fix. I'm always amazed when someone can make beet juice and kale taste delicious. As far as supplements go, I take protein, fiber, and greens supplements in a shake every day no matter what, usually for breakfast. It helps me reach my nutritional requirements as my day gets busier."
> —RAINE MAIDA, SINGER, SONGWRITER, OUR LADY PEACE

1 WHOLE, UNPROCESSED FOODS. Whole foods—those with little to no processing—are essential to living a healthy lifestyle. This includes fruits, vegetables, legumes, whole grains, and cold-pressed oils. Because they've not been stripped of nutrients, whole foods provide your body with the fuel it needs to perform at its peak. Protein-rich nuts, seeds, and amaranth, for example, build cells, hormones, enzymes, and neurotransmitters. The phytonutrients, antioxidants, vitamins, and minerals found in berries, leafy greens, and mushrooms protect your body from free radicals and chronic disease. Cold-pressed oils contain omega-3, -6, and -9 fatty acids, which reduce inflammation, increase cell integrity, feed the nervous system, balance blood sugar, and protect the heart.

A diet filled with these health-enhancing foods will strengthen your well-being and improve your looks, stamina, and focus. Processed foods, however, have been refined of their nutritional value and then enriched with synthetic substitutes. Why strip away naturally occurring nutrients only to add back fake alternatives? To maintain a longer shelf life. While it's fine for a Twinkie or Snickers bar to stay on store shelves for an eternity, it's not okay for the toxins used to preserve them to remain in your body. The rule is that if it can stay on the shelf for months without going bad, it can stay in your body for months, too! Food is meant to be ingested, nourish cells, and then be excreted after its value has been used.

Most processed foods are also formulated with hydrogenated fats, preservatives, food dyes and colorings, artificial flavorings, high-fructose corn syrup, monosodium glutamate (MSG), or refined flours and sugars—ingredients that have been directly linked to diseases like obesity, diabetes, cancer, Alzheimer's disease, asthma, attention deficit disorder (ADD), and cardiovascular disease.

HARM REDUCTION TECHNIQUE: GO FOR THE COLD ONES

Switch to cold-pressed oils when possible, because the fats are not denatured from the high heating methods. Flax, hemp, walnut, sunflower, and argan oils are fantastic-tasting oils that work well drizzled on soups, salads, and vegetables or blended into smoothies.

Because these manufactured, empty-calorie products are high in sugar and nearly devoid of nutrition, they leave you hungry soon after consuming them. This leads to overeating as your body is starved of proper fuel. In fact, did you know that most overweight people are undernourished? No one, rock stars like you included, can sustain clear energy and sharp focus with a body that's undernourished.

These days there are a lot of products in grocery stores that look healthy but are really not. The fastest way to tell if a food will support your nutritional needs is to read the label. If you can't pronounce most of the ingredients, don't eat it. If in fact you are what you eat, does looking like hexamethylene tetramine or tert-butylhydroquinone or polyoxyethylene monostearate sound sexy?

2 Organic and local. Organic foods are an excellent insurance policy for your health. By investing in high-quality ingredients now, you'll reduce your medical costs for chronic diseases in the future. Thinking of organic food as "medicine" makes sense: organically grown foods contain much more vitamins, minerals, nutrients, antioxidants, and fiber than conventionally produced crops, which are treated with pesticides, herbicides, hormones, and other toxic chemicals that promote disease. (Not to mention, organic food tastes better.) What should never be on your "cheat" list? Substandard meats, especially ground beef. The commercial meat and dairy industries treat animals with hormones and antibiotics that in turn end up in the eggs, bacon, and milk we consume.

HARM REDUCTION TECHNIQUE: LEMON AID
If you can't find organic produce, squeeze a little fresh lemon on non-organic fruit or vegetables. Fresh lemon juice draws out pesticides.

Rage Against the Machine
Non-organic foods may also be exposed to irradiation, a process that uses ionic radiation to destroy microorganisms that could be harmful if ingested. It does this by breaking the bonds of the DNA found in viruses, parasites, bacteria, and insects. But when

the bad stuff is zapped, so is the good—the DNA in wholesome, living foods is damaged, which delays their ripening and sprouting, a side effect that benefits businesses because produce lasts longer on shelves. Unfortunately, while irradiated foods are promoted as healthy and nutrient-rich, we don't yet know the long-term of effects of irradiation on our body.

Similarly, genetically modified organisms (GMOs) and genetically engineered (GE) foods contain genes transferred to them from another organism—such as viruses, bacteria, plants, or animals—in order to enhance their benefits or increase their resistance to toxins like herbicides. We're not that far from seeing mind-boggling GM and GE combinations: bananas that have fish genes or eggplants with virus genes or cows with human growth genes. It sounds scary because it is. The Center for Food Safety reports that our grocery store shelves are stocked with GE foods:

- 85 PERCENT OF U.S. CORN IS GE;
- 88 PERCENT OF COTTON, USED TO MAKE COTTONSEED OIL, IS GE;
- 95 PERCENT OF SUGAR BEETS IS GE;
- 91 PERCENT OF SOYBEANS IS GE.

What makes these numbers even scarier is that the foods mentioned above are the basic ingredients for countless processed products. In fact, it's estimated that 70–80 percent of all manufactured foods—from "healthy" cereals, chips, and crackers to soda and lunch meats—contain GE ingredients.

Born in the USA

If you can't find organic products, then locally grown or raised fruits, vegetables, and meats are a great alternative. Native populations have long believed that nature provides us with the nutrition we need within our local areas. These foods may not be 100 percent organic, but they're usually lower in pesticides and hormones than their conventional counterparts you'll find in large grocery stores. And enjoying farmer's markets is a smart way to know and support your local producers and be directly connected to the sources of what you eat.

Look, I'm a realist. I know that many people have limited exposure to healthy food, especially organics, in their area. I also understand that high-quality ingredients can be extremely expensive. Here's the compromise: When shopping for your home, try to buy organic, local, or whole, unprocessed foods 90 percent of the time. Save the other 10 percent for restaurants, parties, vacations, and other situations where it may not be possible or it may just be unsociable.

3   **GOSSIP IN THE GRAINS.** If you've already completed the RxStar Remedy Detox, you've eliminated gluten—a protein found in wheat, rye, spelt, and barley—from your diet. You may incorporate gluten back into your diet sparingly, but limit your servings to one to two per week. If this sounds impossible, I can promise you, it's not. I once toured with a band whose lead singer had celiac disease, an autoimmune disorder that results in gluten intolerance. Management decided to make it a "gluten-free tour" for the entire band and brought in a special catering crew to prepare all snacks and meals. You can imagine the grumblings at first, but by the end of the schedule, everyone lost weight and felt incredible. I say, if they can do it, so can you!

4   **COOL BEANS.** Legumes are high in protein, nutrients, and fiber, but low in fat, making them the perfect vegetarian substitute for meat. They're excellent for restoring kidney and adrenal gland functions, lowering cholesterol, regulating sex hormones, enhancing brain and body development, and regulating blood sugar, water, and metabolism. It's true, cool beans can be not so cool in some situations. To ease digestion (read: gas production), soak legumes in water for twelve hours and change the water one to two times before cooking. Sprouting legumes provide maximum digestibility, amino acids, and enzymes. If you're using canned varieties, rinse them with water before eating. Chew them thoroughly and pair with greens or nonstarchy vegetables. Consider avoiding them when you're in situations where you're not near a restroom, as in trains, planes, and automobiles. Here are some easy ways incorporate legumes into your diet:

BEANS adzuki, anasazi, soybeans, garbanzo, kidney, string, navy, red, black, white
HUMMUS OR BEAN SPREADS choose brands with no added salt, sugar, oils, artificial flavorings, or preservatives; you should be able to pronounce the ingredients, such as lemon juice, olive oil, and garlic
LENTILS brown, green, red, black
PEAS black-eyed peas, chickpeas, split green peas

"If you don't eat your meat, you can't have any pudding."
—*THE WALL*, BY PINK FLOYD

5 I recommend cutting back on animal protein, but if becoming vegetarian or vegan isn't for you, try eating lamb or wild game, which are "cleaner" meat options than beef or pork. Regardless of quality, red meat should always be consumed moderately because of its link to a variety of health conditions, including heart disease, cancer, and diabetes. Avoid eating red meat, pork, and all cured meats during the detox, but beyond that you can enjoy the following in limited quantity:

ORGANIC, GRASS-FED, AND LOCALLY RAISED BEEF OR LAMB

NITRATE-FREE LUNCH MEATS AND SAUSAGES (ALSO KNOWN AS "UNCURED")

WILD GAME SUCH AS VENISON, RABBIT, OR BUFFALO

HARM REDUCTION TECHNIQUE: MARINATE YOUR STEAK

When you marinate red meat for about 30 minutes before cooking, the fats and proteins break down, making the meat more digestible. Try using apple cider vinegar, lemon juice, wine, or tomato juice as a marinade. If you don't have time to marinate meat before cooking, some spices and vegetables also aid in digestion and naturally rid the body of the saturated fats and toxins, including: leafy greens, cabbage, broccoli, onions, ginger, garlic, and marjoram.

6 Healthy fats, including oils, are a very important part of every diet. They produce energy, provide insulation, regulate body temperature, strengthen cell membranes, protect organs and tissues, and transport nutrients like vitamins D, E, A, and K. The key, however, is knowing the difference in quality of the fats you're consuming. Here is the skinny on the best ones to eat:

COCONUT OIL for cooking

COLD- AND EXPELLER-PRESSED VEGETABLE, NUT, AND SEED OILS for dressings and flavoring

EXTRA-VIRGIN OLIVE OIL for cooking on low to medium or to use as a dressing

FLAVORFUL OILS use almond, argan, hazelnut, hemp, and walnut oils as dips or finishing oils for flavor

FLAX OIL one tablespoon of flaxseed oil daily has mega omega-3 benefits so drizzle it on vegetables or add to smoothies

ORGANIC BUTTER not when detoxing and used sparingly other times

7 **DRINK TO THAT.** What you drink is just as important as what you eat for staying focused and energized. The options below contain few to no toxins, such as sugars and harmful additives, but are loaded with antioxidants, nutrients, and other hydrating benefits.

COCONUT WATER make sure to buy 100 percent raw, organic, and unpasteurized

EMERGEN-C mix with water for a vitamin boost

FILTERED WATER use carbon-block or reverse-osmosis water filters

GLASS-BOTTLED SPRING OR FILTERED WATER stay away from plastic-bottled water

NATURAL SODAS WITH JUICE in limited quantity,

they're a healthier substitute for ordinary sodas, but they're not water!

ORGANIC, FAIR-TRADE COFFEE 1–2 cups daily when not detoxing

ORGANIC FRUIT AND VEGETABLE JUICES look for cold-pressed, unpasteurized versions. They have a shorter shelf life but contain live enzymes that are beneficial to your body.

ORGANIC HERBAL AND GREEN TEAS most herbal teas are metabolized as water and may be drunk as a water substitute, and each individual herb has its own nutritional benefits.

HARM REDUCTION TECHNIQUE: SAY NO TO PLASTIC

Keep bottled water to a minimum, especially those stored in #1 or #2 plastic, which seeps toxins into liquid when light hits it. Trade Styrofoam and plastic for stainless steel and glass containers and bottles. And remember, labels don't lie: many brands are simply filtered tap water.

8 **SUGAR BLUES.** If you're detoxing, stick to stevia. Otherwise, keep a variety of the sweeteners listed below on hand rather than artificial sweeteners, which should always be avoided regardless of what color packet they come in. Your best bet is to use natural sugars from whole foods like fruits, vegetables, and grains, in moderation.

Amazake
Barley malt

Date sugar
Fresh fruit juices
Fruit syrup
Molasses: sorghum or Barbados
Organic coconut sugar
Organic, locally grown raw honey
Organic pure cane sugar
Raw and organic agave nectar
Rice syrup
Stevia
Unrefined cane juice powder

HARM REDUCTION TECHNIQUE: SWEET THING

One of my rock stars despised alcohol, drugs, and coffee, but had a mean chocolate addiction. She insisted it put her in a "sultry mood" for her stage persona, although some of us disagreed with her definition of sultry. Instead of milk chocolate, which primarily contains milk and sugar, we switched her backstage habit to high-quality, organic dark chocolate. Its high amounts of magnesium, caffeine, and phenylalanine increased her endorphin levels, a much healthier alternative to the alcohol shots her bandmates were doing.

9 **SPICE GIRLS.** One of the biggest diet fears my clients have is that healthy meals will be bland and boring. Sure, once you remove sugar, salt, fats, and preservatives, food tastes *different*, but you can easily add dimension and excitement with fresh or dried spices and herbs. Life is too short to eat boring food! Here

are a few simple ways to enhance the flavor of your foods:

BLACK OR WHITE PEPPER adds a great kick to almost anything.

FRESH OR DRIED ORGANIC HERBS AND SPICES mint, cilantro, garlic, ginger, basil, rosemary, turmeric, oregano, thyme, sage, and parsley are incredible antioxidants, readily available, and simple to incorporate into everything from smoothies to pasta sauces.

GRAY, PINK, BLACK, OR WHITE SEA SALT sea salt contains more beneficial minerals than standard table salt.

10 **CONDIMENT KINGS.** Most commercial jarred spreads should be avoided during the detox and also when you're maintaining your healthy eating plan because of their added sugar, salt, and oils. Even some organic brands are guilty of this, so read ingredient lists carefully. Here are some healthy alternatives:

BALSAMIC AND APPLE CIDER VINEGAR vinegar is a true health food and is thought to help aid digestion, decrease glucose levels, and lower cholesterol.

ORGANIC KETCHUP organic ketchup contains as much as 60 percent more lycopene, a cancer-fighting antioxidant, than conventional brands. It also typically contains less salt and sugar.

ORGANIC MAYONNAISE look for brands made with

olive and coconut oil, rather than soybean or canola oil.

ORGANIC MUSTARD the healthiest versions have few ingredients: mustard seeds, apple cider vinegar (not distilled), sea salt, and organic spices.

ORGANIC SALAD DRESSING conventional salad dressings can contain unhealthy ingredients that quickly turn salad into a diet disaster, so if you can't find a healthy option, make your own with olive oil and vinegar or lemon juice.

11 **LIVING COLORS.** Keeping fruits and vegetables on hand makes it easy to whip up salads, stir-fries, and snacks. And by choosing from a variety of brightly hued options, you maximize the amount and type of nutrients, vitamins, and antioxidants you're getting each week. Naturally cleansing and alkalinizing, the best options are organic, locally grown, and in-season, and eaten raw, steamed, or lightly cooked. If organic is not available, choose produce that you can eat without the skin and wash using a fruit or vegetable wash. Get creative with a combination of:

SIMPLY REDS apples, berries, radicchio, rhubarb, radishes, peppers, and tomatoes

GREEN DAY leafy greens such as spinach and kale, artichokes, arugula, asparagus, broccoli, and bok choy

THE BLUES AND PURPLES berries, currants, figs, and eggplant

MELLOW YELLOWS peppers, squash, and star fruit

ORANGE CRUSH apricots, mangos, carrots, yams, sweet potatoes, pumpkin, and persimmons
WHITE onions, cauliflower, ginger, garlic, turnips, white peaches, and mushrooms

12 **ALMOND BROTHERS** (and other nuts and seeds I love). Peanuts and peanut butter are best to avoid or eat sparingly. This is a very high-allergy food and may have traces of a mold called *Aspergillus niger*, which can be harmful to your health. For any nuts you eat, look for raw versions—roasted nuts have less nutrient value and usually contain added oil and salt. It's also important to store nuts with care. Throwing a handful of nuts and seeds in plastic containers and Baggies may be convenient for travel, but for your health? Not so much. The oils in these snacks absorb the toxins in plastic. Keep them in glass and in the refrigerator to maximize freshness (the high fat content in nuts causes them to go rancid fairly quickly). Choose any of the healthy protein sources below to keep rockin' all day long:

RAW NUT BUTTERS almond, walnut, cashew, and macadamia butters make rich, creamy, flavorful substitutes for peanut butter. Just be sure to read labels and watch out for salt, sugar, and additives.
RAW NUTS almonds, pistachios, pecans, Brazil nuts, cashews, macadamia nuts, pine nuts, and walnuts are perfect energy-boosting snacks or salad toppings.
RAW SEEDS pumpkin, sunflower, flax, coconut, and sesame seeds are also excellent sources of protein, vitamins, and minerals.

13   **PHISH AND SEAFOOD.** During the detox, you may have limited your intake of seafood, such as shrimp, crab, and lobster—backstage staples for many bands on tour—because these shellfish contain more toxins than fish do. If so, you may incorporate it back into your diet in moderation after the detox, as long as it's wild-caught. Farm-raised fish, the kind most Americans buy, doesn't contain omega-3 fatty acids because these fish aren't eating algae. Choose from the list below and be mindful of your preparation—fish offers the most nutrition when it is baked, broiled, steamed, or sautéed lightly with olive oil.

WILD-CAUGHT FRESH FISH   cold-water salmon, halibut, sea bass, tuna, mackerel, sardines, flounder, and cod are rich in fatty acids and protein. Wild lake and river fish, such as orange roughy and trout, are also healthy options.

WILD-CAUGHT CANNED FISH   albacore tuna, salmon, mackerel, anchovies, and sardines with no added salt are easy additions to salads, pastas, wraps, and rice cakes.

FRESH SHELLFISH   mussels and clams are inexpensive choices that pack as much protein as lean meat; due to their higher toxin levels, shellfish should be avoided during the detox and limited after that; crustaceans (crab, lobster, and shrimp) are less of a concern.

See the guide by Seafood Watch for the best options in sustainable fish that are low in mercury: www.sea foodwatch.org.

14 **WINGS.** Turkey and chicken are often mistaken for healthy choices simply because they're not red meat, but that's not always the case. Many of my rock stars are surprised to learn that the breaded, deep-fried, drive-through options smothered in fat- and sugar-laden sauces are harmful to their body. Most of my clients have switched to turkey, chicken, and eggs purchased from small, local farms that don't use antibiotics, hormones, or steroids. They're higher in protein and nutrients and contain all the essential amino acids. Here's what to look for:

ORGANIC, FREE-RANGE TURKEY AND CHICKEN I suggest baking or roasting for the healthiest preparation. Try not to eat the skin.

ORGANIC EGGS organic eggs come from chickens that are fed a diet free of pesticides, so are lower in toxins than conventional eggs. Try them boiled, poached, or fried in a little olive oil.

WILD GAME our ancestors knew what they were doing when they speared buffalo—wild game meats are great sources of lean protein. And because they typically are killed in the wild, they haven't been treated with hormones or other antibiotics.

15 CREAM (and nondairy alternatives). If you've completed the detox, you've already eliminated cow's milk, a very common allergen, from your diet. Cow's milk is not great for our nutrition or our digestion: pasteurization kills the enzymes that make it digestible, and homogenization allows the buildup of an enzyme called xanthine oxidase, which can lead to arterial scarring. My recommendation is to permanently substitute one of the milk options below, which contain more nutrients and fewer toxins.

ORGANIC COW'S CHEESE AND YOGURT these fermented dairy products are fine for people who have no allergies to cow's milk.

ORGANIC GOAT AND SHEEP CHEESES ounce for ounce, goat cheese packs more protein and calcium and less fat, calories, and hormones than cow's milk cheese. Goat and sheep cheeses are also typically easier to digest than cow's milk cheese.

ORGANIC GOAT AND SHEEP MILK these animal milks are good options for people with an allergy to cow's milk, though they do have a stronger flavor than other milks. You can also find fermented products made from goat and sheep milk, such as yogurt and kefir.

ORGANIC HALF-AND-HALF OR CREAMER when it comes to selecting dairy for your coffee, go for the richer options: organic cream and half-and-half are easier to digest than regular cow's milk.

ALMOND MILK be careful when you shop for almond milk. Believe it or not, some brands contain very few almonds and loads of cane sugar and flavorings. Read the ingredient list carefully and look for "no sugar added" varieties.

RICE, HEMP, AND OAT MILK choose organic brands with no additives or sugar. These options are especially shelf-stable and good to have on hand in your pantry.

SOY MILK look for brands labeled non-GMO and "made with organic soybeans." Avoid soy milk made from "soy proteins" or "isolated soy proteins."

HARM REDUCTION TECHNIQUE: SWAP YOUR CREAMER

Trade the cow's milk in your coffee for organic creamer. It may sound like a strange strategy, but cream comes from the fat of milk, which humans can easily digest. It's the protein molecule in milk, called casein, that we have problems digesting. Pasteurization of cow's milk kills the enzymes that help us to digest the casein or milk protein. Allergic reactions to casein can range from congestion, headaches, fatigue, bloating, and gas to systemic inflammation.

WHAT *NOT* TO EAT: 12 FOODS THAT DERAIL YOUR ROCKSTAR LIFE

There are certain ingredients even Harm Reduction Techniques won't counter if you consume them regularly. Over time, these substances can damage your organs, cause inflammation in the body, and create an environment suitable for diseases like obesity, diabetes, cancer, heart disease, and stroke. Even if you're not detoxing, try to avoid or eliminate the following from your diet:

1 ARTIFICIAL SWEETENERS. You know the ones. They contain aspartame (Nutrasweet, Equal), saccharin (Sweet'n Low), or sucralose (Splenda). Basically, they're chemicals in a pretty little packet. Try natural sugar alternatives like local raw organic honey or agave.

2 OTHER SUGARS. Pour some sugar on me? Probably not after you read just some of the harmful side effects of processed and synthetic sugars and their unhealthy substitutes: diabetes, hypoglycemia, calcium depletion, heart disease, obesity, yeast infections, immune deficiency, tooth decay, neurotransmitter depletion (yes, it affects your brain function, too!), mood disorders, indigestion, premenstrual syndrome and menstrual problems, bone loss, and more. Sugar doesn't sound so sweet anymore.

If you're not sure what to avoid, here's an easy nix list: white sugar, brown sugar, raw sugar, corn syrup, blackstrap molasses, simple sugars ending in "ose" (like fructose, glucose, dextrose, maltose, and sucrose), and sugar alcohols ending in "ol" (such as sorbitol and xylitol).

3 FOOD ADDITIVES, PRESERVATIVES, AND COLORINGS. You really need to be a detective to hunt these down on the ingredient labels, but it's worth it. These are pretty much poison to your body over time: artificial colorings, dyes, and preservatives; fake fats like olestra; MSG (see below); "natural" flavors; hydrolyzed vegetable protein; nitrites, nitrates, and sulfites; and pretty much anything you can't pronounce that more than likely stemmed from a lab, not Mother Nature.

4 PEANUT BUTTER. As we discussed earlier, peanuts are highly allergenic and not the kind of nuts I encourage you to eat. Most peanut butter is filled with ingredients like corn syrup and hydrogenated oils—it's like a tub of peanut-flavored Crisco. If you must eat peanut butter, buy an all-natural variety or go to a store where you can grind it yourself—but try to make the switch to all-natural almond butter.

5 FRIED FOODS. Even the best foods become artery-clogging fat and calorie bombs when doused in oil. No matter how many times you use a napkin to soak up the grease from a batch of onion rings or a cod sandwich, the nutrients buried beneath the batter won't outweigh the bad.

6 HYDROGENATED OR PARTIALLY HYDROGENATED FATS AND OILS (TRANS FATS). Trans fats are found everywhere—margarines, "buttery" spreads, packaged foods. Nothing can make this better. It's like eating plastic. Not to mention they lower good cholesterol (HDL) and raise bad cholesterol (LDL).

7 NON-ORGANIC SOY. Non-organic means it is GMO and irradiated, which basically will turn your cells into a science experiment. Only eat brands that list organic soybeans in the ingredients list. Avoid products with soy protein isolates as well.

HARM REDUCTION TECHNIQUE: TO SOY OR NOT TO SOY

Know the difference between good and bad soy. I once worked with a cross-dressing punk artist who was indulging himself to death with soy products: tofu, cheese, edamame, you name it. He was trying to grow breasts to avoid getting implant surgery. Unfortunately, too much non-organic soy or soy protein isolates can enhance the production of estrogen, which can elevate women's risk of developing certain cancers. I taught him the difference between organic soybeans (the good kind of soy) and GMO soy products and isolated soy proteins (the not-so-good kind). As for enhancing breast size, padded bras work much better!

8 MONOSODIUM GLUTAMATE (MSG). MSG, a salt-like flavor enhancer hidden in most packaged and processed foods, should be avoided at all times. The seasoning has excitotoxic properties—a fancy way of saying it damages nerve cells—and is linked to toxicity syndromes of the nervous system. Some of its negative effects include: headaches, anxiety, fatigue, mood swings, depression, rashes, endocrine problems, attention deficit disorder, insomnia, nervous system disease, and so on. Instead, eat foods flavored with natural salts and/or sea salt. Check ingredient lists and ask restaurants to prepare your meal without

MSG. And check labels for these other code names for MSG:

AUTOLYZED YEAST

CALCIUM CASEINATE

HYDROLYZED PROTEIN

MODIFIED FOOD STARCH

NATURAL FLAVORINGS

NATURAL PROTEIN

SODIUM CASEINATE

TEXTURED PROTEIN

9 **SODA AND SOFT DRINKS.** There is just no nutritive value to soft drinks—they are pure sugar, and have been implicated in this country's obesity epidemic. If you're a die-hard soda fan, try swapping it out for sparkling water flavored with fruit or cucumber, or herbal-infused waters or sodas sweetened with stevia. Otherwise, stick with water and herbal tea!

10 **LUNCH MEATS.** Even if you aren't vegetarian or vegan, avoid lunch meats. If you can't live without your salami or charcuterie, buy brands that contain zero nitrates and nitrites. They may be labeled as "uncured" or "nitrate-free."

11 **ALCOHOL.** This is a tough one, especially when you consider that many people drink an average of 1,000 to 2,000 alcohol calories a day. Spirits are a social lubricant at most business dinners, family functions, and gatherings with friends. Even healthy rock stars are known to throw back a shot before they go onstage to dial up their mojo. If you're a drinker, reduce your alcohol intake by switching to top-shelf brands.

You're more likely to slowly savor a high-quality, more flavorful, and more costly spirit than a low-quality, sugary cocktail.

12 ENERGY BARS. You mean candy bars? There's a fine line between energy bars and savvy marketing that puts a healthy-sounding twist on what's essentially a Snickers. Look for brands that contain at least 10–15 grams of protein coming from hemp, nut butters, whey protein, or pea or rice proteins. The junk to avoid: soy isolates, chemical sweeteners, preservatives, artificial colors or flavorings, casein, which is cow's milk, and anything hydrogenated. Ideally, keep the carb count less than 25 grams. Better yet? Switch to all-natural raw protein bars, which are highly nutritious energy boosters. They contain a few simple ingredients such as nuts, nut butters, seeds, and fruits.

alcohol consumption drastically, but if they "must" drink, I simply give them healthier choices, for example, potato-based spirits such as vodka, juniper spirits like gin, and agave-derived spirits like tequila. These alcohols are mostly gluten-free and more distilled than liquors based on rye, barley, or other grains, so they're cleaner and a little easier on your liver.

Here's a complete list of gluten-free alcohol options:

- Bourbon (corn)
- Champagne (grapes)
- Ciders (fruits)
- Gluten-free beer
- Junmai sake (rice)
- Organic wine (grapes)
- Ouzo (anise)
- Potato-, grape-, or corn-based vodka
- Potato- or grape-based gin
- Rum (sugarcane)
- Tequila (agave)

RxSTAR FOOD SWAPS: USE THESE TO STICK IT TO THE 90/10 RULE

Whether it's pizza or Frappuccinos, we all have foods that we don't want to give up, and we shouldn't have to—indulgence is a normal part of living a balanced lifestyle. However, 90 percent of the time when you're *not* indulging, you can seamlessly substitute ingredients without compromising taste or experience. Below are some of my favorite ways to give clients their food fix without compromising their health:

INSTEAD OF: Sugary, processed candy bars
TRY: Antioxidant-rich, organic dark chocolate

INSTEAD OF: Soy-isolate-packed Luna, Power, or Cliff bars
TRY: Protein or nut bars made with whey, rice, hemp, or nut butter proteins

INSTEAD OF: Traditional soft drinks
TRY: Ginger brew or sodas made with organic juice

INSTEAD OF: Red Bull or other sugar- or caffeine-rich energy drinks
TRY: Green tea or yerba maté

INSTEAD OF: Classic potato chips, like Lay's or Pringles, loaded with salt, oil, and trans fats
TRY: Kettle chips, which contain zero trans fats

INSTEAD OF: Ice cream made from cow's milk
TRY: Dairy-free ice cream made from coconut or rice milk

INSTEAD OF: Hamburgers and fries
TRY: Burritos made with black beans

INSTEAD OF: Milk shakes
TRY: Fruit smoothies made with organic yogurt, nut milks, or raw coconut water

"Health and well-being have become a part of my life. I study a Philippine martial art called Kali, practice yoga, skateboard, swim, paddle-board, walk my dog, and chase my kids around. Additionally, I try to eat as healthy as possible. My meals include fish, chicken, rice, cooked veggies, and plenty of water."

—MIKE MCCREADY, GUITARIST, VOCALS, SONGWRITER,

PEARL JAM

RxSTAR FOO(D) FIGHTERS: OPTIMIZE YOUR LOOKS, STAMINA, AND FOCUS

Now that you know all the great foods in your RxStar arsenal, you can tailor your diet to specific goals. Maximize your looks, stamina, and focus by choosing clean, healthy foods that fight disease, support healing, and fuel a high-performance lifestyle.

Top Foods for RxStar Looks

Looking your best is easier than you think. A diet filled with the following five nutrients will boost your beauty:

ANTIOXIDANTS   reduce free radicals, fortify cell walls, and slow the aging process

GREEN FOODS   act as natural detoxifiers and rid the body of harmful chemicals

OMEGA-3 FATTY ACIDS   strengthen skin and hair, making them more radiant

PROTEIN   builds new cells and helps your body develop lean muscle mass

WATER   hydrates the skin, preventing dryness that leads to wrinkles, and carries nutrients to all of your skin cells

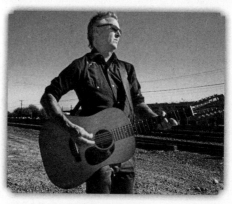

MIKE McCREADY
(DANNY CLINCH)

Some of my favorite nutrient-rich foods for maintaining an ageless look:

Açai
Avocado
Blueberries
Chia seeds
Filtered or spring water
Flax, coconut, and extra-virgin olive oil
Garlic
Greek yogurt
Kale
Lemons and limes
Organic red wine
Turmeric
Wild-caught halibut
Wild-caught salmon

Top Foods for RxStar Stamina

When you increase your stamina, you make it easier for yourself to get through a tough workday or a tough workout. There are five key nutrients for increasing stamina:

1. **PROTEIN** balanced blood sugar = steady energy.
2. **COMPLEX CARBOHYDRATES** these carbs provide lots of ready fuel for your muscles and your brain but burn more slowly than simple carbs, so your hunger won't spike an hour after you eat.
3. **ELECTROLYTES** minerals like potassium, sodium, and magnesium increase endurance by hydrating cells and optimizing energy.

4. **FRUITS AND VEGETABLES** plant-based foods contain phytonutrients that feed the mitochondria—or the powerhouse of our cells—and provide natural glucose for immediate energy.

5. **IODINE AND OMEGA-3 FATS** too much stress leads to adrenal burnout and thyroid problems—the opposite of stamina—so eating foods to support your adrenals and thyroid is key.

Some of my favorite nutrient-rich foods for increasing stamina:

Basil
Black and red beans
Dark chocolate
Fair-trade goji berries
Figs
Lean, organic red meat
Organic green tea or organic fair trade coffee, limited to
    1–3 cups daily
Quinoa
Root vegetables like sweet potatoes and yams
Spinach
Walnuts and hazelnuts

TOP FOODS FOR RxSTAR FOCUS

We've all had days where our concentration was lagging and we felt as though we couldn't quite focus on the task at hand. The food we eat plays a huge role in our mental sharpness. Here are four key nutrients for improving focus:

1. **AMINO ACIDS** these proteins support the function of neurotransmitters like dopamine and adrenaline.
2. **IODINE-RICH FOODS** for thyroid support
3. **FOLIC ACID, VITAMIN B$_{12}$, AND COQ10** each of these is essential for cognitive functions like memory.
4. **PROTEIN** again, it's essential to maintain blood sugar balance so you can keep your concentration on any given task for an extended period of time.

In addition to eating the focus enhancers listed below, avoid refined sugar and wheat products, which lead to brain fog and fatigue:

Beans
Eggs
Flax and coconut oil
Lamb
Licorice or licorice tea
Oatmeal
Oranges
Rosemary
Royal jelly
Seaweed
Wild-caught halibut
Yerba maté

HARM REDUCTION TECHNIQUE: SEA GREENS

Who knew that bento box was also a natural Rx? Seaweed (that green algae stuff you may want to push aside) is a natural detoxifier of radiation and contains nutrients that help regulate your thyroid. Next time you order a sushi roll, grab a side seaweed salad.

COMMON DIET CHALLENGES

You, the rock star, have many lifestyle demands that put you always on the go, whether you're working or playing or traveling. Here are some key lifestyle pointers I use with my clients that will also work for you.

NEVER SKIP MEALS From the second my patients wake up, they're on the go, getting their kids ready for school and activities, hitting the gym, or heading to work early, and don't eat their first meal of the day—maybe a protein bar or a piece of fruit—until late afternoon. Unfortunately, the first meal of the day is also the most important. After not eating all night, skipping breakfast or grabbing doughnuts, bagels, or muffins sets off the day with imbalanced blood sugar. Eating a meal of sugar and carbohydrates without protein is never a good idea, but it's an especially poor start for a day that requires a lot of stamina and focus. By midafternoon, you're even more tempted to turn to more sugar and caffeine to compensate for the energy you didn't get from breakfast. And because skipping meals slows the metabolism, it causes weight gain, fatigue, and mood swings.

"My day never ends. I photograph the musicians on the road and you don't want to miss anything. Everybody sees the fruits of my labor. 'Wow, you were backstage with Eddie Vedder?' And they think that you are just sitting there all night hanging out. But their tour manager's job is to keep them sequestered and let them concentrate on the show. And so I am sitting outside the door. I gotta pee. I'm hungry. But I'm not leaving. So it just compounds itself, and then I just don't end up eating, or I eat badly, or I don't eat at all."

—DANNY CLINCH, ROCK & ROLL PHOTOGRAPHER

KNOW WHEN YOU'RE HALT When you get hungry, angry, lonely, or tired (the acronym HALT), it's easy to turn to addictive foods that contain sugar, caffeine, and refined carbohydrates, which immediately make you feel happier. Unfortunately, this happiness crashes later in the day and sets you off on a roller coaster of energy and mood swings. These quick fixes are mostly empty calories, which can leave you hungry and may lead to binge eating later. Stock your office, gym bag, tote, or carry-on with healthier snack options such as fruit, nuts, or high-quality protein bars so when a craving hits, you don't waste your 90/10 Rule on a vending machine bag of cheese puffs.

YOU BETTER SHOP AROUND

READ THE LABELS OF ALL PRODUCTS Ingredients lists change all the time, so be sure to stay updated on the brands you buy, even ones you've been purchasing for some time. Also, don't trust the brand marketing guys to tell you what's really inside their products. Foods labeled with adjectives like "natural," "healthy," or "wholesome" usually aren't. And all the convenient, prepackaged boxed grains and pastas? They often contain seasonings loaded with sugars and preservatives.

FIND A SHOPPING PARTNER It's easier to stay accountable to your health when you've got someone watching your back. Take a friend or family member with you to shop and you'll spend more time navigating aisles, be more experimental in your food choices, and enjoy the process of discovering new products. Plus they can remind you that a family-size bag of M&M's is not part of your 90/10 Rule.

PLAY WITH NEW CUISINES A RxStar diet isn't filled with iceberg lettuce and flavorless tomatoes. The easiest way to break the misconception that healthy food is boring is to try ingredients and recipes from other cultures and regions. After a trek through a spice aisle, one of my rock star clients discovered a love for Moroccan food and learned a few recipes after the tour ended.

> "I eat more of a Mediterranean diet. One of the things that I learned living in Europe is to eat smaller meals. They eat a lot of figs, olives, fruits, vegetables, and fish. And of course everything has olive oil with it. Sharing and eating off each other's plates is very Mediterranean. I prefer that."
> —GARY LOURIS, SINGER, SONGWRITER, GUITARIST, THE JAYHAWKS

KEEP A POSITIVE ATTITUDE Shopping shouldn't be a chore; it's an opportunity to play with foods and find what you love. This is your life, make it fun! I spent an afternoon on tour with a heavy metal band carousing through natural food stores and non-organic groceries comparing product labels with them. They turned our lesson in learning harmful ingredients into an adventure and created new names for heavy metal and punk rock bands based on toxins in foods. Here are a few they came up with: the Trans Fats, Red Dye #3, the Aspartames, the MSG Effect, Sodium Nitrite, the Irradiators, the Hydrogenators, and Benzoic Acid Test.

4 TRICKS TO READING AN ORGANIC LABEL

Use these simple strategies for locating organics when you shop.

1   **LOOK FOR THE STICKER**   All produce sold in grocery stores contains a sticker labeled with a Price Look-up (PLU) Number, which is standardized by the International Federation for Produce Coding for easy identification. Regularly grown or "conventional" fruits and vegetables have a four-digit number that starts with a 3 or 4. Organic and genetically modified fruits and vegetables have five-digit numbers that begin with an 8 and 9, respectively.

2   **READ THE LABEL, NOT THE NAME**   Watch out for savvy marketing. Only products that are labeled "certified organic" or "certified organically grown" by a state agency or third-party certifier (such as OneCert) can be considered organic. These products will carry the certifier's seal of approval or certification of endorsement on the packaging.

3   **EXAMINE THE LIST OF INGREDIENTS**   Organic products usually have a shorter list of ingredients with names that are easy to recognize and pronounce. When it comes to meat, look for "hormone-free," "antibiotic-free," and "grass-fed," which indicates the animals are eating grass rather than grains. They have higher levels of omega-3 fatty acids and less saturated fat. For chicken and eggs, terms like "free-range" and "organic" mean the chickens are free to roam outside of cages eating local foods, rather than housed in cages, and pumped up with hormones and antibiotics.

4 KNOW WHAT THE TERM "ORGANIC" REALLY MEANS When you see the word "organic" on a label, it refers to the percentage of organic ingredients within the product; for example, "100 percent organic" products must be made entirely from organic ingredients. "Organic" products, however, must contain at least 95 percent organic ingredients, even if each ingredient isn't specifically described as being organic. And the phrase "made with organic ingredients" on a processed food label simply means that the product contains 70 percent organically produced ingredients. "Natural" doesn't mean the same thing as "organic." It's a marketing term that's not regulated by the government but used by brands that know consumers equate the term with healthy.

15 TWEAKS YOU CAN MAKE TODAY TO LIVE LIKE A ROCK STAR:

"I am predominantly vegetarian, but I do eat eggs. I'm sometimes limited in meal options, so I eat lots of veggies, salads, and a carb in the morning. If there is a juicer at a venue, I'm all over it. And I try not to eat too much after the show."
—BRIDGET BARKAN, SINGER, SONGWRITER, SCISSOR SISTERS

1 START TODAY It's important to eat carbohydrates, like rice cakes and fruit, with a healthy protein, such as raw nuts or nut butters, in order to lessen the impact of sugars on your blood sugar levels, keep you feeling full longer, and increase your metabolism. My favorites are a hard-boiled egg with vegetables or a sprouted grain bagel with goat cheese.

SET A GOAL TO Eliminate refined sugars and flour products.

2 **START TODAY** Eat three balanced meals a day. Fasting, or going without eating for as little as five hours, causes your body to secrete cortisol, which causes fat to deposit around your midsection. Too much cortisol slows your metabolism because your body perceives itself as starving, and can also cause inflammatory diseases.

SET A GOAL TO Break meals into five or six smaller meals or snacks, eaten throughout the day.

3 **START TODAY** Prepare all of your meals for the day in the morning so you don't make poor food choices out of desperation when you're hungry or healthy choices aren't available. Lack of planning puts you at risk for eating processed foods or skipping meals.

SET A GOAL TO Keep your pantry, car, and office stocked with healthy snacks at the beginning of the week.

HARM REDUCTION TECHNIQUE: DETOX YOUR DECAF

If you are drinking decaffeinated coffee, choose organic, fair-trade, and water-processed brands to avoid the chemicals used in the extraction process.

4   **START TODAY**   Drink 8–10 glasses of water per day to keep the body hydrated and functioning optimally. Water is the number-one nutritional deficiency in our society. A minimum of 64 ounces is recommended if you live a sedentary lifestyle and don't drink caffeine (for every cup of caffeine you drink, your body secretes 2 cups of water), but some studies suggest that amount be even higher—13 cups for men, 9 cups for women. The best measure is to look at your urine, which should be clear to pale yellow. And if you're performing four-hour concerts like Bruce Springsteen or the Rolling Stones, you'll need much more than 64 ounces a day to make up for fluid loss. Add a cup before you exercise and after to ensure you stay hydrated.

    SET A GOAL TO   Drink filtered water, rather than tap or plastic-bottled, which can contain toxins like fluorine, chlorine, and heavy metals.

5   **START TODAY**   Eat two to three servings of fruit and four to five servings of vegetables in a variety of colors every day.

    SET A GOAL TO   Switch to organic fruits and vegetables whenever possible, and incorporate smoothies or shakes into your diet to maximize servings.

6   **START TODAY**   Eat one to two servings of legumes per day.

    SET A GOAL TO   Switch to organic legumes and soybean products, trying a new variety or preparation each week to optimize nutrient intake.

7   **START TODAY**   Eat one to two servings of nuts per day.

    SET A GOAL TO   Switch to raw, organic nuts or organic nut butters that contain no added sugar, salt, oil, or preservatives in the ingredient list.

8 **START TODAY** Reduce caffeine to 1–2 cups per day to minimize the withdrawal effects and add my Harm Reduction spices (see box) to reduce its acidity.

SET A GOAL TO Incorporate more organic green tea into your diet, which contains less caffeine than coffee and more antioxidants.

HARM REDUCTION TECHNIQUE: SPICE UP YOUR COFFEE

Black tea and coffee are highly acidic—and acidic foods are not good for the body. Having a high acid pH level is linked to gastrointestinal, immune, and circulatory problems. To neutralize some of the acid, add a spice like cinnamon, cardamom, vanilla, chicory, or nutmeg to your coffee and tea.

9 **START TODAY** Switch from refined white flour to whole grains, such as brown rice, quinoa, oatmeal, buckwheat, and millet.

SET A GOAL TO Go gluten-free. Gluten not only causes weight gain, increases fatigue, and reduces concentration, but also has been linked to autoimmune and inflammatory diseases like cancer, celiac disease, rheumatoid arthritis, and diabetes. In addition, gluten affects the opiate receptors in the brain, leading to addictive behavior and binge eating. You'll notice this if you've ever been to an Italian restaurant and found it impossible to eat just one piece of bread.

10 START TODAY   Avoid cow's milk—even fat-free and low-fat varieties—and switch to almond, soy, rice, or other nondairy milks. Pasteurization, a heating process that eliminates bacteria in milk, also destroys the enzymes that allow us to digest milk protein, known as casein. When eaten, this protein causes inflammation that may result in mucous conditions and allergies.

SET A GOAL TO   Eat only organic cow's cheese and yogurt—the digestive enzymes removed by pasteurization are added back in order to ferment and process them. Or switch to goat and sheep dairy products, which have very few hormones and contain fat and protein molecules similar to human milk, making them easier to digest.

11 START TODAY   Limit meat consumption based on your blood type. If you're type O, stop at three to five servings a week. Type A, which is associated with vegetarian diets, should limit their intake to one to two portions weekly. Avoid all processed meats, which contain nitrates and nitrites, preservatives that have been linked to a variety of conditions such as heart disease, cancer, and Alzheimer's disease.

SET A GOAL TO   Eat only organic, hormone-free, and grass-fed meats or wild game, if a vegetarian diet doesn't work for your body type or lifestyle.

HARM REDUCTION TECHNIQUE: MEAT ON THE SIDE
Limit red meat consumption by using small amounts of it as a component of vegetable-rich dishes like tagines, curries, or stews.

12 START TODAY   Avoid processed poultry meats and egg substitutes, such as Egg Beaters, which may contain additives, like flavorings, oils, and thickeners.

SET A GOAL TO   Eat only organic and free-range chicken and eggs, which are more nutritious and contain fewer additives, like hormones and antibiotics, than their commercial counterparts.

HARM REDUCTION TECHNIQUE: YOU CAN HAVE YOUR EGGS—AND THE YOLKS, TOO

A rock star client with high cholesterol refused to give up his favorite food—eggs—and even took cholesterol-lowering drugs, so he could "cheat" and eat them. We agreed that he could continue his egg "addiction" as long as he didn't break the yolks when he cooked them. Keeping yolks intact by boiling or poaching them preserves their lecithin, a naturally occurring substance that breaks down fats and helps to metabolize cholesterol. After using this trick and moving from heavy to moderate egg consumption, my client was able to stop taking his medicine!

"If there is one thing to take for salvation on tour, it's hot sauce! I took hot sauce with me on tour, and I still do, Frank's!! I had to do it to survive. The sad truth is that most meals are catered for everyone to like them and, consequently, they have no taste whatsoever."

—PETER BUCK, GUITARIST, R.E.M.

13 **START TODAY** Eat fish two to three times per week with greens, like kale and spinach, which are natural detoxifiers that help your body release toxins like mercury from seafood.

SET A GOAL TO Consume only wild and sustainable fish, rather than farmed, which contain fewer toxins, are better for the environment, and have more omega-3 fatty acids from eating algae.

14 **START TODAY** Eliminate refined white sugar and high-fructose corn syrup, often found in unexpected places, such as bottled salad dressings, pasta sauces, and granola. Be sure to read labels.

SET A GOAL TO Limit natural sugars as well, by reducing your consumption of honey, agave, and cane sugar.

15 **START TODAY** Eliminate all hydrogenated fats and vegetable cooking oils that are not "cold pressed," a low-heat production process that preserves the nutritional value of the oil. This includes extra-virgin olive oil and cold-pressed nut and seed oils. High-quality fats preserve and strengthen the integrity of your cell membranes. Eating just a couple of tablespoons a day will give you all of the health benefits and still allow you to fit into your skinny jeans.

SET A GOAL TO Take 1 tablespoon daily of flaxseed oil, which contains omega-3, omega-6, and alpha linoleic (ALA) fatty acids, which, studies show, reduce risk of inflammation, high cholesterol, heart disease, and cancer. I prefer the oil over the capsules because it takes thirteen capsules to get the same benefits that you get in one tablespoon of pure oil.

HARM REDUCTION TECHNIQUE: PEEL YOUR PRODUCE

To reduce the impact of harmful pesticides on non-organic produce, avoid eating the skin. An artist I worked with became so terrified of pesticides that he kept a squirt bottle backstage to polish all fruits and vegetables if he couldn't verify whether they were organic. One day I even found his assistant peeling the skin off grapes for him! You don't have to go that far—if the skin or rind isn't removable (or you don't have an assistant to de-skin it for you) don't panic. Simply wash the outside of the fruit or vegetable thoroughly with a produce wash that contains essential oil of lemon, a powerful detoxifier and astringent.

RxSTAR REMEDY ROAD SNACKS

When you're constantly on the go, it's much more difficult to stick to the 90/10 Rule by winging it. Instead, build your healthy lifestyle around how you really live, whether your days include traveling, commuting, or simply rushing between appointments. Below are healthier options for the office, the airport, or the gas station.

FOOD TRIPPING

"I guess you can say that I am a 'foodie.' I also travel a lot.
I may be on the road with bands, for speaking engagements,
for making movies, or just for adventure. I found it extremely
hard to find healthy alternatives to the general fast-food
fare. My business partner, Peter Glatzer, and I developed the
Food Tripping app [at SHFT.com] as a tool for people to find
alternatives to fast food while out on the road. The options
range from healthy, local, and smaller establishments to mom-
and-pop joints and places off the beaten path. This way we can
support the local economy and connect with people that have
unique cultural experiences."

—ADRIAN GRENIER, MUSICIAN-ACTOR-FILMMAKER-ACTIVIST,
WRECK ROOM, HONEY BROTHERS

The Office:

Blue corn chips with fresh guacamole

Goat cheese on gluten-free rice crackers or a sprouted
grain bagel

Hummus or bean dips with cut veggies

Organic vegetable chips (no hydrogenated fats) with
spinach dip made with organic yogurt

Organic yogurt with fresh fruit

Raw food protein bars

Raw nut butters with gluten-, preservative-, and sugar-
free rice cakes or apples

Raw, unsalted nuts with dry or fresh fruits

The Gas Station:

Cheese sticks
Fresh fruit
Glass-bottled water
Granola bars
Greek or plain yogurt
Honest brand iced teas
Nuts and dried fruit
Turkey jerky

The Airport:

Cheese and fruit plates
Hummus and veggie plates
Nuts and dried fruits
Sandwich wraps
Smoothies
Yogurt and granola cups

THE STARVING ARTISTS TOUR

I spent a week touring with a group of fourteen urban hipsters from Brooklyn. They were skinny but beginning to develop the telltale spare tire around the middle, an indication that they were not balancing their blood sugar and were eating a few too many carbs. If you are what you eat, this group would have been 99 percent Crisco and high-fructose corn syrup. They had every soda and energy drink known to man to substitute for the lack of sleep and long hours, along with massive, family-size bags of synthetic snacks. How could they eat like this and maintain any level of sanity? They were truly "starving artists" as they were eating lots of empty calories and getting very little nutrition from the high-calorie foods.

One day, they decided to stop at a "health food restaurant" just off the highway in an attempt to impress me. It was In-N-Out Burger! They proclaimed that the fries were made daily from freshly cut potatoes, which gave them the status of being healthy. That crossed the line! The next afternoon, I took them on a field trip to Trader Joe's and taught them how to shop for truly healthy, convenient foods, which were packaged yet free from nearly all hydrogenated fats, additives, high-fructose corn syrup, and colorings. They were also impressed that the healthy food was actually cheaper than most of the junk food! The band was thrilled with the variety of options and the flavors.

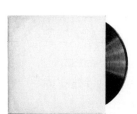

BONUS TRACKS

"Since switching to a mostly vegan lifestyle, we feel a lot more energetic and more open. In a word, I'd say 'lighter.' However, when we're on tour, we're not militant about it, but still don't eat meat and just do the best we can with what's offered. You can locate a burger anywhere, but it's crazy hard to find an organic apple in the middle of America!"

—SHARE ROSS, BASSIST, **VIXEN**

"I follow a very strict diet while on and off tour with Moon Hooch. We eat healthy, local, vegan on a budget while we are touring across the U.S. We even create our own recipes. I do not consume any animal products at all and try to have a steady intake of green superfoods and fresh fruits. I incorporate as much organic food in my diet as possible and consume only whole grains."

—MIKE WILBUR, SAXOPHONIST, **MOON HOOCH**

"I started taking things out of my diet little by little and discovered that I was healthier. I was not just physically healthier but mentally much sharper. I am not for being on a diet. I am just for changing your diet in the little ways you can. Make small adjustments. You don't have to be a superfreak. I'm not a superfreak diet guy . . . yet."

—BEN JAFFE, **PRESERVATION HALL JAZZ BAND**

"I drink as much water as absolutely possible; I drink a lot of coconut juice that is raw, not the Pepsi Cola, Vita Coco kind of stuff, but the good stuff. I make the promoters go and get that for me when I am on tour. "

—COURTNEY LOVE, SINGER, SONGWRITER, MUSICIAN

"Eat to live. We are machines. Would you feed your car cow anus and salt? NO. It would run like shit. You are what you eat."

—STEVE LUKATHER, GUITARIST, **TOTO**

THE ROCKSTAR REMEDY

"My doctor told me this tip and it seems to work: Drink as much water as you're drinking caffeine and alcohol. After every cup of coffee, have one cup of water. The same goes for drinking. So that's what I do."

—A. JAY POPOFF, SINGER, SONGWRITER, DRUMMER, LIT

"At some point on tour I became a vegetarian. Then I became a vegan.

Both decisions were based on ethics as well as awareness. Unfortunately, I gravitated toward a lot of processed and sweet vegan foods. It took me a while before I realized I was fooling myself with bad results. Ultimately a balanced whole-foods, mostly plant-based diet worked for me. But I was plenty unhealthy along the way thinking that I was healthy!"

—MIKE D (DIAMOND), RAPPER, SONGWRITER, DRUMMER, AND PRODUCER, THE BEASTIE BOYS

"You know it is really all in the portions, portions, portions. Instead of eating this huge footlong submarine, just split it with somebody. When I was traveling with British bands, I would bring them to the New York delis. They would see the size of the sandwiches and say, "Are you kidding me, man? In England that would feed a family of four!"

–KRAIG JARRET JOHNSON, GUITARIST, KEYBOARDIST, SINGER, SONGWRITER, THE JAYHAWKS, GOLDEN SMOG

"I think people should step back when they are looking at food and try to make a good decision about what they eat. You eat a salad every day and a piece of fruit and it will make a world of difference. You can still have your other foods that you like, but a change like that with vegetables and fruit is the best for you and your body."

—STEVE RILEY, DRUMMER, **LA GUNS**

"I'm my biggest fan. And if more of us were our biggest fans, we would take better care of ourselves. I gluttonize on life."

—**LYDIA LUNCH**, POET, SINGER, PERFORMER, ACTRESS, AUTHOR

CHAPTER 8

STAGE THREE: ROCK STAR BODY

Y ou've detoxed, implemented some new healthy habits, and learned to eat like a rock star, so now it's time to rock your body! In this chapter, I'll share my exercise regimens, body treatments, and beauty tricks that will have you looking and feeling at the top of your game.

Exercise is important for countless reasons, but the main ones that are essential to fueling a demanding lifestyle are: energy/stamina, strength, flexibility, and stress relief. You need energy and stamina to perform at your best, juggle a variety of obligations, excel at your job, be a great parent, and find time to do all the things you want and need to do. You need strength and optimal health to play just as hard as you work and truly enjoy life. You need flexibility to prevent injuries of the muscles and joints while you are on the move. Flexibility is the key to longevity. When you are flexible and free in your movements, your internal organs are working great and not stagnant. Flexibility of the body also promotes a flexible and serendipitous attitude of the mind, which keeps you open to life's experiences without cynicism. And finally, you need exercise for stress relief and an outlet for all the pent-up energy and frustrations that come with daily living. The stress reduction that comes with exercise is one of its most powerful benefits.

> "I thought a lot about it, how I looked. I liked the idea of not looking like what was expected, what was supposed to be rock—what was out of context to the kind of music we were playing. Sort of going against what Sonic Youth sounded like, the band's expectations, and, you know, wearing something that was just feminine looking, you know. I never wanted to be rock hard. I never wanted to be super muscle-y like Madonna, but I wanted to be strong."
> —KIM GORDON, BASSIST, **SONIC YOUTH**

Unfortunately, you don't have the luxury of spending all day perfecting your body. Neither do rock stars. The trick is to maximize your downtime and make every minute of activity count. Here is my philosophy for creating real change that lasts:

- **DO WHAT YOU ENJOY.** You're busy enough as it is, so adding something pleasurable that you look forward to each day will be its own reward. And you're more likely to stick to it in the long run and be present and passionate in the moment.
- **DO WHAT WORKS FOR YOU.** You've got your own interests, time issues, money situation, and more, so what works for someone else might not be ideal for you. Try things out. A regimen that's ideal for you today may take too much time or be less stimulating tomorrow. Maybe you'll say this is my groove for a few months, but now I'm bored. There's nothing wrong with that. Test-driving different activities stimulates neurons to create new connections, so the more you experiment, the

healthier you become. The key is finding a good fit for your life in this moment.

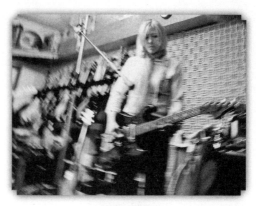

KIM GORDON
(DANNY CLINCH)

- **DO WHAT YOU CAN, WHEN YOU CAN.** Gyms, personal trainers, and fitness classes are a modern luxury. You don't have to have a health club membership to be a fit person. Nor do you have to spend hours every day working out. That isn't practical for all lifestyles, nor is it necessary for your body to stay in shape. The key is to do the most you can for your body whenever you get the chance. Make movement a mindset and a lifestyle. Find every area of your life where you can sneak in activity, from walking to the train or office to dancing while you make dinner, garden, or do housework. Remember that cardiovascular exercise has cumulative benefits so every few minutes you incorporate into your day—a quick flight of stairs up to your apartment or a personal rave to your favorite music in your living room—adds up.

"I go to the gym every single day. Whether it's a light, moderate, or heavy workout is not important. Consistency is the key. That I'm there in some way every day. Even the mildest, lightest workout benefits me. The key is to have a positive outlook."
—DAVE NAVARRO, GUITARIST, JANE'S ADDICTION

Do get up and move!

I prefer the terms "movement" or "activity" rather than "exercise" or "fitness." When combined with flexibility, they are two of the keys to longevity. It's not just movement and flexibility of the body, but also of your mind and spirit, because they help you deal with changes and transformations that are normal parts of being human and living your life. When you stop moving, changing, and adapting, you become stagnant, stuck, and rigid. Your physical body breaks down; you become mired in the past and stop moving forward.

> **"Playing drums for two hours a day helps keep my girlish figure! I clipped an odometer to my shoe as an experiment once . . . and after a show it said 12.3 miles! There's my daily exercise right there!"**
>
> —TOMMY LEE, FOUNDING DRUMMER,
> **MÖTLEY CRÜE** AND **METHODS OF MAYHEM**

Rock stars are the perfect example of people who stay flexible with their workout routines. On days when they travel, the only exercise many of them get is walking through airports or carrying their bags. You can probably relate. If your schedule is similar, take stairs instead of the escalator or walk between gates, rather than use moving walkways. Stretch on flights or between bus stops. It's about being creative within your lifestyle and circumstances and staying inspired to be as healthy as you can most of the time. It's been estimated that Mick Jagger runs, walks, or dances around twelve miles per concert. If you need motivation, strap on a pedometer and calculate your steps walked throughout a normal day. You may surprise yourself. Carrying this little tool also keeps exercise at the top of your mind, so you stay inspired to take the long way home or even the stairs.

THE BENEFITS OF EXERCISE AND MOVEMENT

Musicians know that exercise is brain *and* body food—physical activity doesn't just build a beautiful body; it also creates a high-performance mind. It reduces stress, clears their mind, and gives them time and space to focus on themselves. Studies show that many forms of exercise also improve cognitive function, heighten creativity, and strengthen neural connections, particularly those that are coordination-based like tennis, table tennis, choreographed dance, and other sports that require hand-eye coordination. And you thought progressive companies were just putting in gyms to help workers release stress. Turns out all your hot dance moves also improve your mind. How? Physical activity:

- boosts endorphins (your body's natural painkillers),
- builds muscle that in turn increases metabolism and calorie burning,
- enhances brain function,
- enhances cell function, which improves longevity,
- facilitates your body's use of nutrients from food,
- increases circulation of blood and lymph, which helps detoxify your body,
- kick-starts production of neurotransmitters (serotonin and dopamine),
- oxygenates cells, which aids the anti-aging activities of the body, and
- relieves stress in minutes.

Basically, exercising is like cleansing your blood and purifying your organs every day.

Countless studies have also shown that staying active and flexible reduces your risk for countless diseases, trims your waistline, and enhances your looks by increasing circulation and flushing toxins.

EXERCISE AND MOVEMENT

Each form of exercise and movement provides specific benefits and meets certain goals of the RxStar body. Aerobic exercise supports energy by oxygenating the tissues through the circulation of blood and nutrients throughout the body. Aerobic exercise is great for building endurance and strength of the lungs and heart as well. It can also enhance immune function. Examples of aerobic exercise include running, swimming, biking, walking, and dance classes. Strength training provides support for the musculoskeletal system by integrating balance and alignment into our postures. Examples of strength training are weight lifting, Pilates, circuit training, and some forms of yoga. Flexibility forms of exercise support the return of the muscles to the natural resting state and open the body from a contracted state. They also are supportive to the alignment of the structure of the spine. Yoga, stretching, and martial arts are forms of exercise with a focus on flexibility. All forms of exercise have the potential to relieve stress and enhance the body-mind connection. It is essential that your weekly exercise and movement rituals and routines incorporate aerobics, strengthening, flexibility, and stress reduction methods.

FITNESS REGIMENS

Cycling

Cycling is the perfect metaphor for health because you simply get on the bike and take off for an adventure. The road is your canvas to create a new experience every time you exercise. If you're in an urban area, you're saving gas, easing your commute, and exploring your neighborhoods. Those outside of cities usually benefit from a rougher terrain and a more meditative experience in nature. Stationary bikes are fine as well, although they don't have the scenic component. But you can do it while you're watching a movie or catching up on the news. So if that is what gets you moving, no problem.

"One of the benefits of living in New York City is the culture of the street. People walk everywhere. But I live in Brooklyn, so I ride my bike all over the place. I struggle with a bit of depression, so if I'm like wanting to sort of stay inside under my bed, I'll force myself to get on my bike. It's enough motion that it propels me into the city. Then when I'm in the city, I end up having some kind of adventure."
—JOSEPH ARTHUR, SINGER, SONGWRITER, GUITARIST

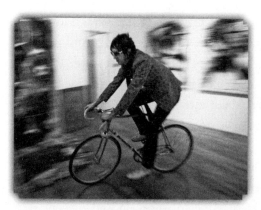

JOSEPH ARTHUR
(DANNY CLINCH)

Dance

What is more natural than moving to music? This is the number-one activity for rock stars and their fans. The time artists spend onstage is their exercise for a day. While many musicians stretch or warm up before a show, their main workout is the performance, which is mostly dancing. You don't need to hit a concert, club, or studio to get your fix. Nearly every genre from salsa and Zumba to belly and ballroom dancing offers routines online for free or low monthly rates. It's available whenever the mood strikes or you have time to kill. Have your own personal rave in your living room.

Martial Arts

Martial arts, a favorite practice among many musicians, is a discipline that not only strengthens and stretches muscles, but also works with Qi or the vital life energy, aligns and uses energy to heal, improves coordination, and focuses the mind. The variety of types is endless, from kung fu to tai chi, and the fun is in trying new experiences. The practice is also special in cultivating the teacher or master/student relationship as well being part of a dojo or workout community.

Running

Running looks like pure torture to me, but many of my artists love it because it's a powerful stress reliever (thank you, endorphins), it's a complete full-body workout when you use proper form, and you can do it wherever you are, so it's a great form of exercise for people who travel frequently. Make sure you're wearing supportive shoes and getting enough electrolytes. I recommend eating a banana, and having one or two Emergen-C packets or some coconut water to enhance electrolytes and prevent dehydration from intense sweating. Start with minimum stretch sessions of ten minutes before and after running to warm up and prevent sprains and strains.

Strength Training

You don't get rock star abs and arms without a little strength training. It's a great option for those with busy lives because you can follow simple routines that can be done in gyms or hotel rooms, at home, and, yes, even on tour buses. Weight machines work well, but you can find effective moves that use your body weight or elastic resistance bands to give you an equally fantastic workout. I highly recommend lifting for extra-flexible people who need to strengthen muscles, boost their metabolism, or kick-start weight loss after they've plateaued. This can be a major part of a rebuilding plan if you've gotten injured or need to gain bone density. If you're not familiar with the weight room, work with a trainer for a session or two to make sure you get the proper technique and a customized program that uses all of your muscles and incorporates flexion and extension. We want your body to be balanced. Again, be sure to stretch before and after.

Swimming and Other Water Sports

Swimming is an excellent option for people with injuries who shouldn't be doing any weight-bearing activities. Water adds a natural resistance that increases muscle tone in a gentle way. It's aerobic and calming at the same time. Remember to stretch before and after—just because you feel less resistance in the pool doesn't mean your muscles aren't working. Post-swim, rinse the chlorine off your skin and eat some seaweed salad or some dried seaweed snacks. Seaweed naturally protects your thyroid from chlorine exposure, which can wreak havoc on your thyroid gland by displacing the iodine.

Many rock stars, including Jack Johnson, are big-time surfers. You're competing with yourself and nature, and enjoying the meditative experience of the ocean. Not to mention it takes incredible core strength and coordination to maneuver the board. Other water sports such as kiteboarding, bodyboarding, kayaking, and canoeing are ways to enjoy Mother Nature and get some exercise, too.

Walking

Walking is an underrated fitness activity and is the one we have the easiest access to. Walking at a brisk pace can be aerobic and enhance endurance. It is an easy way to kill two birds with one stone, too. Walk while you run errands. Walk to work. Walk with friends instead of meeting for coffee. Get yourself a pedometer and it may motivate you to take the stairs and walk places you would normally drive to.

Yoga

Many artists are naturally drawn to yoga for its fusion of mind, body, and spiritual components. What we know as modern yoga in the United States is mainly the branch known as "hatha," which includes several styles of physical practice using postures, or asanas. The practice is only one limb out of an eightfold path of living that includes meditation, eating healthy, and other disciplines. The purpose of the asanas is to clear physical interference in the body so our mind and spirit will be more clear and aligned. When first starting out, get into some of the alignment-based types such as Iyengar and YogaWorks with a well-trained instructor so you can familiarize yourself with the postures, especially if you have injuries. These will teach you how your body should be in each posture. Ashtanga, vinyasa, and other power yoga styles typically involve more movement and are often referred to as flow yoga. It's a fantastic option for those looking for a more athletic and aerobic style of workout.

MEET THE 90/10 RULE OF FITNESS

There's no one-size-fits-all cure when it comes to fitness: no certain class, no miracle program, no fat-burning elixirs, no exact number of hours required, no proven prescription that works for everyone.

That's the good news, because this means the perfect program for you is one you can adapt to your lifestyle, one that you are willing to perform most days. You want something (or a series of somethings) that you can commit to 90 percent of the time.

Exercise moves on the same spectrum of health as other areas of your life. Some weeks or months, you're dedicated and never miss a goal. Other times, work, family, or social obligations get in the way of your commitment. Don't beat yourself up when you can't work out every day. That's normal. That's life.

8 THINGS TO ASK YOURSELF WHEN BUILDING A FITNESS ROUTINE

"Sometimes I'll just turn on music and dance. I love music and dancing and singing and it's all about the stuff you love. There's no excuse for not exercising. I've gone on Pinterest and found workout boards with videos. Just do something, even if you can't commit to thirty minutes. You always feel better knowing that you at least tried, even if you only squeeze in ten minutes."

—EVE JEFFERS, AKA EVE, GRAMMY AWARD–WINNING RAPPER-SONGWRITER AND PRODUCER

- **WHAT DO I LOVE TO DO?** Think about what activities you love and what you'd look forward to doing in your free time. If you dread cardio machines, don't expect yourself to log several hours a week on one.

- **WHAT FINANCIAL RESTRICTIONS DO I HAVE?** If a gym membership or personal training isn't in your budget, take up a sport that won't break the bank: running, walking, biking, hiking, or swimming. Or, if you love group classes like yoga, dance, and Pilates but can't find a good deal, look for online streaming options that range from cheap to free. You can do the routines on your schedule.

- **WHAT TIME RESTRICTIONS DO I HAVE?** A lot of my clients have erratic hours or don't leave work until after the gym is closed. Online classes are also a great option for those who like instructors or need motivation. Or, multitask: While you're watching TV, stretch or use the balance ball, treadmill, or stationary bike. People always make time for TV, so why not burn some calories at the same time? Same strategy works when socializing. If you're meeting a friend for coffee, take it to go and walk a few laps at the park. Go dancing with friends. Do like singer-songwriter Holly Miranda and carry a Frisbee in the car—she tosses it with her band at rest stops while touring.

- **WHAT'S MY EXERCISE STYLE?** Do I prefer a regular routine? Do I work on the pendulum? Or am I completely erratic?

  Follow your own natural rhythms. If you know you can't commit to same time, same place for your daily workout, don't sign up for classes only to skip them. Or, if you need the structure of a set schedule, create one and do what it takes to keep it. Enlist friends, give yourself incentives. Or if you're completely erratic, find an activity that you can do on the fly and carry your cross trainers with you. Many musicians tour with equipment and gear so they can squeeze in a workout when space opens on their calendar.

- **WHAT HEALTH RESTRICTIONS DO I HAVE?** If you've got temporary considerations—for instance, you're pregnant, doing a detox or cleanse, or recovering from a back injury—then choose an exercise that is supportive for you during this restricted time.

- **WHAT HEALTH CONDITIONS DO I HAVE?** Consider where your body is on the spectrum of health. Perhaps you have a heart condition and your cardiologist has ordered some aerobic exercise for you. Or maybe your doctor has prescribed yoga and walking to treat migraines or stress headaches. Many musicians have repetitive stress injuries from years of playing instruments and lugging gear on the road. Those with joint or back pain, for example, often find relief trying low-impact sports such as swimming, yoga, Pilates, or biking. Those experiencing fatigue or depression often benefit from higher-intensity, full-body workouts that engage their mind and bodies, boost endorphins and serotonin, and require focus—they spend less time on negative thoughts and learn to stay in the moment. Don't give yourself an excuse to quit. Instead, work where you're at now and evolve your routine as you get stronger and healthier.

- **DO I NEED FORMAL CLASSES AND TRAINERS TO MOTIVATE ME OR AM I SELF-MOTIVATED?** No matter how cool or effective the hottest new trend, you won't stick with a program if the format or style doesn't fit your personality. If you need a drill-sergeant-style boot camp to get up and moving, a treadmill or DVD workout won't likely do the trick. But if you're the Iron Man type, the idea of the latest, greatest Spinning classes probably isn't as exciting as tearing it up on the open road. Working out in a group may inspire a little competitive fire or it may be a distraction, depending on your level of fitness. Align activities with what brings out the inner athlete in you, so you feel the rush that comes with pushing yourself and achieving a goal.

> "After my last tour, I really got into Pilates, and that's probably been a good thing to keep up on tour, since all you need is a DVD and maybe a yoga mat if you feel fancy."
>
> —NINA ELISABET PERSSON, SINGER, **THE CARDIGANS**

- **HOW ACTIVE IS MY LIFE IN GENERAL? AND HOW CAN I BALANCE WHAT I DO IN MY JOB OR DAILY LIFE WITH A FITNESS REGIMEN THAT ROUNDS THINGS OUT?** You don't have to be a rock star to log loads of miles during the course of a normal day. In fact, your normal routine may already include a lot of movement. For example, landscapers, mail carriers, and real estate agents typically move all day long. Or perhaps you have an office job, but you bike or walk to work. Consider your natural activity level when customizing a new workout.

After you've taken into consideration how you live each day, use exercise to balance your routine. For instance, studies show that as many as 80 percent of roles in today's job market are sedentary or include only light activity. If you're in that camp, you'll likely enjoy the release of more aerobic or intense workouts. People with stressful jobs benefit from yoga, which gives them a mental release. Rockers like Dave Ellefson, Ori Kaplan, Jordan McLean, and Bridget Barkan make yoga a regular part of their routine because their shows often involve a great deal of cardio.

Those on the opposite end of the spectrum—contractors, landscapers, or others with more physical careers—would benefit from less intense activities like yoga, swimming, or stretching. If you feel lonely or isolated during the day, as freelancers, telecommuters, or new moms often do, try an activity that engages you socially, like dance. Perhaps your daily routine isn't that challenging or stimulating. If so, competitive sports or workouts that involve choreography stimulate the brain.

Finally, if you're already working out, consider adding exercises that balance your dominant nature. For example, flexible people tend to love yoga but could enhance their body by incorporating more strength training. Runners and weight lifters tend to be stiff and usually don't like stretching, but stretching would benefit their body by balancing it more.

Some of the best exercises for those living a RxStar lifestyle tend to be those that can be done anywhere and incorporate a mind, spirit component. I've listed a few here that are favorites of my clients and indicated why they may fit into your lifestyle, too. Remember, health is an adventure. Sometimes it takes experimenting before you find your thing.

CREATE-YOUR-OWN FITNESS ROUTINE

What should your regimen look like?

To get the most bang for your health buck, exercise should:

- Be aerobic—getting your heart rate up enhances the function of the circulatory and respiratory systems;
- Be fun and enjoyable so you're focused in the moment and stick with it in the long run;
- Engage body, mind, and spirit so you work out harder, stronger, and ultimately better (that means greater results!);
- Improve flexibility to help prevent injury and improve endurance and performance;
- Include a warm-up to increase blood flow to muscles and gradually get your heart rate up, as well as a cooldown to get your heart rate back to normal, stretch the tightened

muscles, and clear the lactic acid from your system that makes you feel sore.

- Strengthen muscles, which increases spine stability and boosts metabolism so you burn more fat and calories;

How much do you need?

DAILY: I recommend 30 minutes minimum of basic movement or activity, like taking the stairs instead of the elevator, walking at lunch, or taking a leisurely bike ride on a Sunday afternoon. This will give you all the brain and body benefits you need for a fit mind, body, and spirit. Again, that's not gym time, that's activity. Walking at a good clip and stretching are important every day at a minimum to keep blood flowing, maintain flexibility, and prevent injuries when you get to more intense workouts. For example, I walk three miles a day just moving between my patients' rooms. Find little ways you can be more active in your day.

WEEKLY: Now that you're up and moving every day, incorporate RxStar fitness:

- Add 30 minutes of aerobic activity 3–5 times per week.
- Add 30 minutes of strength training 2–3 times per week.
- Integrate mind, body, and spirit practices at least 1 time per week.
- Incorporate a warm-up and cooldown before each session.

This can be as simple as walking on a treadmill, doing some easy yoga poses, or using the foam roller to ease tight muscles before you work them.

RxSTAR TREATMENTS: REJUVENATE YOUR BODY

If you're giving out more energy than you're taking in, you're bound to feel depleted from time to time. The treatments I'm sharing with you in this section are designed to facilitate your recovery and recharge your energy, no matter how hard you push yourself. Then not only may you have energy to get through your day in a happy and productive way, but you may also extend beyond your limits and live like a rock star. You will see an improvement in your life socially and creatively and physically. You will gain the vitality that comes from balancing your health with enjoying your life.

The remedies I recommend focus on the physical body by aligning the spine and releasing muscle tension and stress. They also enhance the energetic balance of the body by working on the nervous system and meridians. The effects that these treatments have on the physical and energetic systems of the body will in turn benefit you emotionally and spiritually.

The way this plan fits with your lifestyle is much the same. It maximizes your energy, improves physical performance, increases endurance, reduces risk of injury from repetitive stress or wear and tear, and helps healing of physical and structural problems. This plan will help to recharge your adrenal glands, nervous system, and endocrine system by restoring your vital life force, or Qi. The endocrine and nervous system are like our batteries. This may give you the extra oomph to push beyond normal activities. Prolonged travel, working overtime, commuting, and stress may drain you and your life force and add additional stress to your physical body. These therapies will help you to restore and regenerate so that you are not running on empty.

The part of our nervous system known as the autonomic is responsible for all the automatic functions of our body such as digestion, immunity, breathing, heart activity, circulation, and much more. This "autonomic nervous system" has two particular divisions or modes of operation:

1. Parasympathetic mode, aka "rest and digest." In this mode we are able to rest, relax, restore, and regenerate.
2. Sympathetic mode, aka "fight or flight." In this mode we are energized, focused, concentrating, and ready to deal with stress.

The treatments I recommend specifically affect the nervous system and allow your body to go into the parasympathetic or "rest and digest" mode. Modern life has most of us in sympathetic overload and we are in this state of "fight or flight" for prolonged periods of time due to constant stress, unhealthy relationships, excess work, overbooked schedules, and so on. If you don't take an equal or greater amount of time to rest and regenerate, then over time your batteries will wear down. I like to use the metaphor of a car. You can have a car that is moving, stopped at the light but the engine is still running, or turned off. If the car turns off you can fill the tank with gas and recharge the batteries. Most of our nervous systems are like the car that is driving or the one that is at the light but the engine is running. We are never turning "off." This in turn will cause the adrenal glands, endocrine system, and nervous system to wear down, since you cannot charge the batteries and fill up your tanks with gas. This syndrome is also known as "wired and tired." It can manifest as fatigue, anxiety, insomnia, overwhelm, irritability, depression, and other stress-related symptoms.

If you push the envelope and live life to the fullest, you're likely in this category. In fact, 70 percent of my non-rock-star clients operate in the "wired-and-tired" category: moms, business executives, students, workaholics, and fun-aholics. Most people who fall out of a natural rhythm of work and activity followed by rest and repair will end up depleted if this continues long enough.

The treatments in this section help to facilitate your nervous and endocrine systems to go into that rest, recharge, regenerate, and repair mode. This enables and equips you to handle the extra stress of your RxStar lifestyle. Incorporate these treatments into your life regularly for the best results. This is ideal because maintenance and prevention are the best insurance policy. At the very least, use these therapies when you are feeling depleted and burned out to help you get back in the game and repair.

While some may resonate with you more than others, it is great to try them all at some time on your healing adventure!

1. Chiropractic Manipulation—Realign Your Spine and Structure

Spinal realignment provides a foundation for bodywork techniques and a platform for physical activities and exercise. Aligning your spine and skeleton improves the function of your muscles and nervous, circulatory, and lymphatic systems. It may also improve organ function related to certain neurological regions. Chiropractic emphasizes how the structure of the body and spinal alignment affect the function of other systems. Your initial session will include an orthopedic and neurological assessment with postural analysis of your musculoskeletal system. The practice places emphasis on the functional integrity of the body and how it correlates with the other aspects of health. Your doctor will apply manual manipulation to the spine and extremities to realign structure, promote physical functions, and stimulate the nervous and vascular systems. Stretching and muscle balancing techniques help maintain the alignment longer. These include massage, physical therapy, yoga, and strength training.

Not surprisingly, along with massage, chiropractic is the most popular backstage support. In fact, chiropractors and massage therapists are typically the first to travel with bands because they're the most useful supporters of this lifestyle and heal the things that cause the spine to go out of alignment, cause back pain, and create stress on the body. Although you may not be performing in front of tens of thousands of screaming fans or stage-diving off a boardroom table, you may experience similar wear and tear from daily repetitive activities, like computer use or carrying a heavy bag on your shoulder.

The RxStar Remedy Rx:

- **INJURIES:** 1–3 times per week until acute phase is over
- **MAINTENANCE:** 1 time per week or monthly, depending on activity
- **A BUDGET-FRIENDLY OPTION:** stay aligned with yoga and stretching and supplemental visits at the clinics of chiropractic schools

2. Massage and Bodywork—Relax Your Muscles

Massage and soft tissue therapies relieve muscle spasms and stress, increase circulation of blood and lymph, improve muscle and skin tone, detoxify tissues, and promote overall well-being. Many of the varieties and styles can help you stay relaxed and stress-free, but they can also be used to treat pain or a specific injury. I typically recommend Swedish massage, deep tissue massage, acupressure, shiatsu, Thai massage, or Tui Na. My clients never complain when I recommend massage or bodywork, and it is by far the most popular backstage treatment at concerts and music festivals.

The RxStar Remedy Rx:

- **INJURIES:** 1 time per week
- **MAINTENANCE:** 1 time per month
- **A BUDGET-FRIENDLY OPTION:** rather than luxury spas, visit massage schools or Chinese acupressure salons in larger cities

3. Reflexology—Relieve Your Feet

This is not your ordinary foot rub. Reflexology is a deep-pressure-point massage of the feet and hands that stimulates reflexes associated with different organ systems. An entire map of your body can be laid out in just your hands and feet. This map shows the correlation between the reflex points and other parts of your body. Reflexology helps stimulate organ function, relaxes your feet and entire body, reduces stress, and clears your mind. This is a perfect treatment for people who wear high heels or platform shoes, especially if they're on their feet all day. I would often be doing reflexology treatments on tour buses between different cities as this is an easy and effective treatment to do, with no tables or oils necessary.

The RxStar Remedy Rx:

- TRY AT LEAST ONCE
- 1 TIME PER MONTH WOULD BE HEAVENLY!
- **A BUDGET-FRIENDLY OPTION:** massage schools or DIY reflexology. Many books and online references include guides on performing basic techniques at home.

4. Rolfing—Restructure Your Fascia

Also known as "structural integration technique," Rolfing is a form of bodywork that releases and manipulates the fascia, which is the connective tissue surrounding muscles, bones, and organs. It has a reputation for being very painful but in recent years the methods have become more tolerable and enjoyable. Rolfing is excellent for people with postural problems such as scoliosis, hunchback, and swayback. I frequently recommend Rolfing for people with injuries in which the scar tissue has started to create problems with joint mobility and flexibility such as "frozen shoulder syndrome" and "whiplash." But certainly, if you are not happy with your posture, you travel frequently, or you find yourself slouching over your desk or computer, then a Rolfing series may be just the right thing to change the entire way you carry yourself. It's something I suggest to nearly all of my rock star clients, who often experience structural problems from bending over instruments and slouching in plane and bus seats for hours on end.

The RxStar Remedy Rx:

- SERIES OF 10 SESSIONS 1–3 WEEKS APART BASED ON THERAPIST RECOMMENDATION

5. Cranial Sacral Therapy—Reset Your Nervous System

Cranial sacral involves the gentle manipulation of the cranial bones of your head, cervical spine, and sacrum with the intent of aligning the autonomic nervous system and bringing you into the parasympathetic mode. This mode helps you relax, restore, regenerate, and rest. The technique works by releasing the tension of the membranes covering the brain and spinal cord, also known as the meninges. The meninges connect the nervous system and skeletal system and in turn improve the flow of cerebral spinal fluid, blood, and nerve energy. Based on very gentle touch, this therapy can be performed on anyone and results in profound relaxation.

I find this therapy to be extremely helpful for treating headaches, sinus problems, anxiety, insomnia, chronic stress-related conditions, ear or jaw pain, and post-traumatic stress. It has also proven to be one of my favorite remedies for rock stars recovering from drug or alcohol addiction or suffering from anxiety and insomnia.

The RxStar Remedy Rx:
- AS NEEDED OR A SERIES OF 1 TIME PER WEEK FOR SPECIAL CONDITIONS

6. Acupuncture and Traditional Chinese Medicine—"Rebalance" Your Energy

Acupuncture falls within Traditional Chinese Medicine (TCM), a health system that's several thousand years old and also includes therapies such as Chinese herbal prescription, cupping, moxibustion, and Tui Na massage. During a treatment, fine sterile needles are inserted into specific points called acupuncture points, which are basically little vortices of energy. These points are found on meridians, or energy channels, mapped out throughout your body. Qi is the vital life-force energy that flows through these meridians. Each meridian is associated with a particular organ system. The points all have particular effects on balancing your body and may relate to specific physical, emotional, or spiritual imbalances. In general, acupuncture is beneficial for almost any disharmony of the body and mind because it's a complete system of medicine of its own. The points chosen are the best ones determined to recalibrate and rebalance the energy of the particular person at that time.

The benefits of acupuncture in a hectic lifestyle are endless. I've used the technique to treat clients recovering from addiction, reducing cravings, lessening withdrawal symptoms, combating anxiety and depression, bolstering creativity, improving sleep, relieving pain, eliminating constipation, alleviating headaches, stopping smoking, and beating jet lag, fatigue, and insomnia. Acupuncture can be used alone or in conjunction with another therapy, such as chiropractic, herbs, and massage as part of Traditional Chinese Medicine.

The RxStar Remedy Rx:

- ADDICTION: 1–7 times per week
- PAIN: 1–3 times per week
- HEALTH CONDITIONS: 1 time per week
- MAINTENANCE: 1 time per month for energy tune-ups
- BUDGET-FRIENDLY OPTIONS: tai chi or qigong practices or local acupuncture school clinics

Acupuncture Add-Ons:

If you deal with any of the issues below, ask your acupuncturist to add additional points to the basic treatment. Or you can press the same points with your fingers and get some acupressure benefits. Some of the favorite acupuncture points for rock stars include:

ADDICTION—5-NEEDLE AURICULAR PROTOCOL FOR ADDICTIONS

Alcohol—liver 3, large intestine 4

Fatigue—Du 6, stomach 36

Hangovers—stomach 44, Ren 12

Headaches—large intestine 4, Du 20
Heartache—Ren 17, heart 7
Heartburn—Ren 12
Insomnia—Yintang
Laryngitis—San Jiao 5
Motion sickness—pericardium 6
Pain—large intestine 4
Sugar cravings—spleen 6, stomach 36

RxStar Beauty: Look Forever Young

Physical beauty is our inner balance, vitality, and health radiating outwardly. The skin and hair in particular are influenced by the proteins, fats, vitamins, and minerals that we eat, drink, and absorb. I see this reflected in my clients after they have completed the 21-day detox. They look ten years younger with radiant, glowing skin and hair.

Three of the biggest beauty poisons and age saboteurs: sun exposure, chemicals in products, and smoking.

Here Comes the Sun

Sun worshippers know that there are many physical and emotional benefits to ultraviolet rays. When full-spectrum sunlight hits your retina, it stimulates the pineal gland to produce a hormone called melatonin, which regulates your body's hormones and natural rhythm cycles. Melatonin enhances your mood and improves sleep quality by increasing serotonin levels. Increased melatonin and serotonin production also lessens carbohydrate cravings and increases testosterone and sexual vitality. You need just twenty minutes of sun exposure per day without your sunglasses to get the benefits.

Another important benefit of sun exposure is activation of vitamin D, which can only be absorbed through the body via exposure to sunlight. You also need about 20–30 minutes of sun exposure per day on the skin itself for the activation of vitamin D, which enhances mood, immune function, and hormone balance. During this time, you should not use sunscreens. For the remaining time you spend outdoors you should use a nontoxic sunscreen to protect yourself from too much radiation. And, yes, cloudy days count, too.

However, as we all know, too much of a good thing is harmful—exposure to UV rays can cause premature aging, skin damage, and skin cancer.

Healthy sun worship checklist:

✔ Get 20 minutes of sun per day without sunscreen or sunglasses.

✔ Get vitamin D levels checked by your doctor.

✔ Wear sunglasses with UVA protection.

✔ Wear a hat or sunglasses and use shade for excess sunlight.

✔ Use sunscreens that meet Environmental Working Group (EWG) guidelines and ratings.

✔ Choose broad-spectrum sunscreens with SPF between 15 and 30, and reapply every two hours and/or after swimming or sweating.

✔ Use mineral-based zinc oxide or titanium oxide sunscreens, which are more effective than chemical-based varieties.

✔ Take omega-3 oils before and after sun exposure. As a general recommendation, take 1 tablespoon of omega-3 or flaxseed oil daily.

✔ Avoid burning and remember that incidental sunlight (nondirect exposure, such as sitting in the car on a sunny day) can also cause sun damage.

✔ Get skin moles and marks checked regularly by a dermatologist.

Chemical Overload

Your skin is your largest organ, and it absorbs a large percentage of what you apply to it, for good or for bad. What you put *on* your body goes *into* your bloodstream, so choose personal care products that contain all-natural and organic ingredients. The Environmental Working Group website's Skin Deep section is a great resource for choosing the safest, best skin-care products.

Avoid these chemicals in skin, hair, and nail products:

- AMINOPHENOL
- BENZALKONIUM CHLORIDE
- BRONOPOL
- BUTYLATED HYDROXYANISOLE (BHA)
- DIAMINOBENZENE
- DIBUTYL PHTHALATE (DBP)
- DMDM HYDANTOIN
- FLUORIDE
- FORMALDEHYDE OR FORMALIN
- FRAGRANCE
- HYDROQUINONE
- METHYLCHLOROISOTHIAZOLINONE
- METHYLISOTHIAZOLINONE
- OXYBENZONE
- PARABENS (PROPYL, ISOPROPYL, BUTYL, AND ISOBUTYLPARABENS)

- PEGs (POLYETHYLENE GLYCOLS), CETEARETHS, AND POLYETHYLENE
- PETROLEUM DISTILLATES
- PHENYLENEDIAMINE
- PHTHALATES
- RESORCINOL
- RETINOIC ACID
- RETINYL PALMITATE AND RETINOL (VITAMIN A)
- TOLUENE
- TRICLOCARBON
- TRICLOSAN

HARM REDUCTION TECHNIQUE: NO SWEAT!

Avoid using antiperspirants or deodorants with aluminum. Excess aluminum in the blood can have a number of ill effects and has even been linked to Alzheimer's disease. Antiperspirants also prevent sweating, which is one way the body eliminates toxins. It is not a good idea to stop toxins from being released near the breast tissue. Use organic and natural deodorants that are free from aluminum. Essential oils can also work well as natural deodorants.

Cosmetic Acupuncture: An Alternative to Botox

One of the trendiest, but potentially toxic, beauty fixes for anti-aging is Botox. Only recently have some rock stars and other celebrities spoken out against its side effects and potentially dangerous long-term use. A healthier first line of defense is what I call the Acupuncture

Facelift, a safe, all-natural, and nontoxic alternative to cosmetic surgery and Botox. Cosmetic acupuncture uses the ancient wisdom of acupuncture along with nutrition and lifestyle changes to transform your appearance from the inside out. This is true anti-aging therapy that enhances your beauty by harmonizing your overall health.

Some of the benefits of cosmetic acupuncture:

- BALANCED HORMONES
- DECREASED PAIN
- IMPROVED SLEEP
- IMPROVED SKIN TONE OF FACE AND NECK
- IMPROVED UNDER-EYE APPEARANCE
- INCREASED ELASTICITY AND MOISTURE IN SKIN
- INCREASED ENERGY, VITALITY, AND SENSE OF WELL-BEING
- REDUCED ACNE AND SKIN INFLAMMATION
- REDUCED WRINKLES
- SOFTENED SMILE LINES
- STRESS REDUCTION

Plastic surgery is another option for looking young for ages; however, there are alternatives to try before you go under the knife. Remember that imperfections make us unique and give us character. We don't want to look like everyone else, do we?

Plastic Surgery Alternatives Checklist:

- ✔ Add the detox shake to your morning routine
- ✔ Drink water, water, water, and more water
- ✔ Exercise daily and incorporate yoga into your regimen
- ✔ Fill your diet with fresh fruits and veggies and organic omega-3 and -9 oils

- ✔ Get more fresh air
- ✔ Get regular facials and massages
- ✔ Try cosmetic acupuncture
- ✔ Use organic skin care for face and body

THE BOTOX TOUR

One band in particular had no interest in any of my naturo-pathic remedies to improve their health, other than passive treatments such as massage and stretching before going onstage. Changing their diet or using natural remedies was not their thing. That is, until they realized how well the natural therapies helped you heal from plastic surgery.

Their tour had convenient breaks for the artists to have anti-aging cosmetic surgery support. This was their answer to years of self-destruction and the war against gravity. This band did it all: Botox, face-lifts, tummy tucks, lip injections . . . the list goes on. Natural remedies, which we used at every stop on the tour, can be exceptionally helpful for supporting the post-surgery experience by decreasing bruising, reducing inflammation and swelling, and healing connective tissue. I also recommended lymphatic drainage massage and other soft-tissue therapies to minimize the side effects of their plastic surgery work.

I was quickly elevated to "genius" status when one artist's plastic surgeon told him that he had never seen someone heal so quickly from surgery. *Whatever you are doing*, he said, *is working brilliantly*. The good news is that this opened him and the other band members up to the fact that, "Hey, the snake oil really works!" By the end of the tour, they were all on anti-aging diets and supplements and getting acupuncture facelifts for the spots where the Botox injections had failed. Sure, it's sort of funny how they came around to believing in natural medicine, but I am just happy they did.

Argan Oil: The Moroccan Fountain of Youth

One of my trade secrets is argan oil, the Moroccan fountain of youth, which I recommend to all my clients. This multipurpose anti-ager is derived from the argan tree of Morocco and has been used for centuries for its numerous culinary and medicinal benefits. In the beauty world, this oil is coveted because of its high level of essential fatty acids, including linoleic acid, which protect and repair skin and hair. Argan is also loaded with vitamin E, one of the most powerful antioxidants in neutralizing free-radical production and protecting cell membranes from lipid peroxidation. Put simply, it's excellent at slowing the aging process of the skin and enhancing its natural beauty. This is why is it sometimes referred to as "liquid gold."

A true beauty elixir, Argan oil also:

- IMPROVES SKIN ELASTICITY
- MOISTENS DRY, ITCHY SCALP
- MOISTURIZES THE SKIN
- PROMOTES SCALP HEALTH TO RESTORE HAIR GROWTH AND VITALITY
- PREVENTS SPLIT ENDS
- PREVENTS STRETCH MARKS
- REGENERATES AND REJUVENATES AGING SKIN
- REPAIRS DRY, BRITTLE NAILS
- RESTORES LIFE AND SHINE TO HAIR
- SLOWS THE APPEARANCE OF WRINKLES
- SOOTHES AND RELIEVES SKIN DAMAGED BY SUN AND SMOKING

Smoking

My advice in a word: STOP.

If you must smoke, here are my Harm Reduction Techniques for minimizing the toxic impact of cigarettes:

- LIGHT UP WITH MATCHES INSTEAD OF KEROSENE LIGHTERS.
- ROLL CIGARETTES WITH CELLULOSE PAPERS.
- SWITCH TO ORGANIC AMERICAN SPIRIT TOBACCO—MOST CIGARETTES ARE FULL OF CHEMICALS IN ADDITION TO TOBACCO AND NICOTINE, BUT THESE CIGARETTES ARE "CLEANER."
- TRY CIGARS INSTEAD, WHICH ARE MADE WITH PURE TOBACCO ROLLED IN TOBACCO LEAVES. They are also so rich and heavy that you need less to get the same effect.
- USE ORGANIC TOBACCO AND ROLL YOUR OWN TO SLOW YOU DOWN AND MAKE THE SMOKING MORE CONSCIOUS.

Your Stop-Smoking Checklist:
- ✔ Start with a detox, followed by a healthy diet
- ✔ Balance blood sugar
- ✔ Balance neurotransmitters through supplements. Contact a doctor through neurorelief.com for guidance.
- ✔ Exercise daily to give yourself a different source of energetic high

- ✔ Schedule acupuncture sessions
- ✔ Try hypnosis with a licensed practitioner

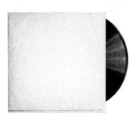

BONUS TRACKS

"I'm sixty-one and I play with a band called the Slim Kings who are between twenty-five to thirty-five years old. I can still kick their asses! During my thirty years with Billy Joel, I was called a musical athlete. During a single show, I burned twelve or more calories per minute. I still play like it's the last time I'm ever going to drum. I wouldn't be able to do this if I weren't in top health."

—LIBERTY DEVITTO, DRUMMER, **SLIM KINGS, BILLY JOEL**

"People think that rest and just staying in stationary places can benefit someone having a bad back. But it couldn't be more the opposite. You have to find the appropriate level of resting and action, and movement to help."

—TRAPPER SHOEPP, SINGER, SONGWRITER, GUITARIST,
TRAPPER SHOEPP AND THE SHADES

"I practice jow ga kung fu, a martial arts hybrid that combines beauty and self-defense. These exercises not only strengthen but also work the internal energies, or chi, and they are choreographed so that you can apply them to dance or physical activity. The practice helps maintain focus and flexibility so that you can flow from situations that are bleak to moments that are meditative and help find solutions. I always believe that the physical release of stress will create flow or a pathway to peace."

—AMAYO, SINGER-DRUMMER,
ANTIBALAS AFROBEAT ORCHESTRA

"I teach 5Rhythms dance workshops. That's where I get my highs from, rather than external things like food, drugs, or alcohol. The 5Rhythms workshops are a joy, not hard work. Meditation is hard work. Sitting there with your own mind and trying to get beyond it . . . that ain't easy for me. But dancing, I'll do that any day. Give me that one."

—TIM BOOTH, SINGER, JAMES

"I love running but not on the streets or in the canyons. I'm all about the stationary machines in the safety of the gym! I'm not trying to break nuthin', get bit by nuthin', chased by nuthin'—friend of mine says, 'Let's go to Runyon Canyon,' and I say, 'Huh? There's dogs and snakes and crazy Hollywood people, no, thanks!' Put me on a treadmill! Here's my recipe for happiness: Keep it simple and safe. Don't push the envelope if you don't have to."

—ERNIE CUNNINGHAM, AKA "ERNIE C," GUITARIST,
BODY COUNT

"I do have to deal with back issues, as a lot of musicians do. The two things that were a revelation for me were yoga and massage therapy. Yoga helps not only my back issues but also with my general mental state. These days, yoga studios are everywhere, so it's not hard to find them in whatever town we are in."

—PAT SANSONE, WILCO

"I pulled my back out back in '84 with WASP. What worked was a good stretching routine every morning for fifteen minutes. I don't have back pain anymore because of this. Even people without bad backs should do this, as it is great for the entire body to be fully stretched out before you start your day. I do try to stretch at all stops on the road, and on flights."

—STEVE RILEY, DRUMMER, LA GUNS

"When we do our routed tours we hire a network of massage therapists in cities around the country. I always seemed to be on the table during Nugent's set, so now anytime I hear 'Stranglehold,' I experience an eerie calm."

—KEVIN CRONIN, SINGER-GUITARIST, REO SPEEDWAGON

"When we get into the tour bus, it is like being in a submarine. You get a lot of light and sensory deprivation. It is important to make sure you get enough sunlight. For me, I try to run or walk a little bit every day. Seeing the sun is good for the mental thing."

—CRAIG FINN, SINGER, HOLD STEADY

STEVEN TYLER'S ADVICE ON HOW TO FIND A GOOD SURGEON:

"Find out which physicians have been sued in the last five years. And which physicians have done the most operations. Then you go to the top four, and before you leave their office, you ask them, "If you were having this operation, who would you recommend perform the surgery?" And if they give you the name of one of the top three doctors you just saw, you mark them 'keepers.' "

—STEVEN TYLER, SINGER, MULTI-INSTRUMENTALIST, AEROSMITH

"I quit smoking when I was twenty-seven. I smoked a pack and half a day before that. That is when I really started running. It burns off a layer of mental fog and depression. I try to run about four to five miles per day. It is a great way to explore the neighborhood at home and on tour. Maybe I'll see a cool record store and go back there when I have my wallet. That's cool."

—CRAIG FINN, SINGER, HOLD STEADY

"We have been going to the Lin Sister Herb Shop in Chinatown. You go in, they look at your eyes and your tongue, they feel your pulse, and they ask you questions. Then they combine the herbs and make a specific brew for you. I also get acupuncture there. It's reinvigorating and there are no side effects. Like you know every medication you take that you hear on television. Right? The herbal teas are completely affordable and they are the best thing for you. For everyday treatment and maintaining your health, I swear by Chinese medicine."

—STEVE JORDAN, DRUMMER, GUITARIST, COMPOSER,
MUSICAL DIRECTOR, AND PRODUCER

"I don't mind the lack of sunlight. It probably has something to do with growing up in England until I was eight. Or maybe because I've spent most of my life either inside nightclubs or in dark recording studios in basements, which are great in case of an air raid but not necessarily for vitamin D intake. Personally, I don't need sunlight, but I realize my body probably does, so I try to go outside in the day as much as I can."

—MARK RONSON, ARTIST, DJ, PRODUCER, AMY WINEHOUSE, LILY ALLEN, BRUNO MARS, SIR PAUL McCARTNEY

"It's an athlete's journey, being on the road. As a performer, you're actually burning the kind of calories that an athlete is burning for an hour and a half a day, and then you're being social after that. So musicians are athletes that smoke and drink."

—JENNIFER FINCH, BASSIST, L7

"I started to do Pilates when Coco was born, because I got horrible back pain from bending over and picking her up, carrying her, breastfeeding, whatever. So I started to do some Pilates and, later, yoga. I have picked up many different injuries over the years from all the wear and tear of carrying the bass and jumping around and playing, and I was never convinced the yoga was helping the issues, I was never feeling, 'I am doing the right thing,' so I kind of backed off from that. So now I am looking for a dance class! I am at a crossroads."

—KIM GORDON, BASSIST, SONIC YOUTH

CHAPTER 9

STAGE FOUR: THINK LIKE A ROCK STAR: DON'T ACT YOUR AGE!

We've talked about how to nourish your body with food and exercise, so now it's time to revitalize your mind and spirit and recharge your batteries to keep you looking and feeling forever young.

If you've already achieved your physical goals through diet and exercise, you've probably noticed that you're feeling better mentally, too. Healing the physical body can give you the strength to deal with emotional issues, like stress, grief, or trauma. At the same time, managing issues like worry, fear, loneliness, or anger can have a positive impact on your hormones, nervous system, immune system, and energy levels. When mind, body, and spirit work together, you move toward optimal health.

At the core of my philosophy is the *free spirit* mind-set. It's the willingness to embrace all the ways you can heal yourself with an open mind and adventurous attitude.

Rock stars are the quintessential free spirits. They're young at heart, no matter how many decades they've been touring or what the age on their driver's license says. They freely experience life in the moment and choose to create their own reality. That's why many of them, even in their seventies, seem ageless. They're not conforming to preconceived notions that "this is what happens at this particular age" or "this is how I should act at a certain age." They're living proof that mental and spiritual components of medicine are just as critical to fantastic health as your physiology.

A lot of artists are drawn to alternative practices because they want to find deeper meaning in life or experience a stronger connection to a power greater than themselves. The following practices will help you free up your own rock star spirit so that you can live more fully in the moment, recapture your zest for life, and get to that childlike essence within you where agelessness can be unleashed. Try one or more of them and see which ones work for you, your belief systems, and your lifestyle. Again, there's no perfect Rx that is right for everyone. There are too many varieties of people for there to be only one right path. As Gandhi said, "There are many paths up the same mountain." The emotional and spiritual remedies must resonate for you in this moment and give you a sense of openness, serenity, and nonjudgment. This is your adventure, so enjoy it!

MEDITATE

As mentioned before, there are a number of meditation styles, but in general, the practice is a way of clearing your mind. It's a quiet time to reflect, a space when you aren't thinking negative thoughts or, if they arise, you're gaining greater awareness of them in a nonjudgmental way.

It can bring clarity, a focus on the present, and enhance your sense of connection to nature and people. There are many physiological benefits to meditation that have been researched, such as lowered blood pressure, decreased inflammation, reduced stress, improved sleep, enhanced energy, strengthened immunity—they're endless. Some studies show that just twenty minutes a day equals anywhere from two to six hours of sleep per night. This can be very useful for a rock star on a sleep-deprived tour schedule!

I recommend transcendental meditation (TM), a style that takes just twenty minutes twice a day and is a favorite among my clients. Although I've practiced a variety of meditation techniques from around the world, I found this to be very easy to incorporate into my daily life and the results were phenomenal: within two weeks, I felt more relaxed and peaceful, less reactive, more accepting, more forgiving, and more playful. And I didn't have to stop other forms of meditation, relaxation, or spirituality to practice TM.

PRAYER

I think of prayer as talking to our higher power and meditation as listening to our higher power. There are as many types of prayer as there are people. It can take the form of reading from a spiritual text, reciting a mantra, giving thanks and gratitude, expressing love, or just sending a blessing. For those who are opposed to the idea of this practice, consider it as positive thinking. We can't think about two things at the same time. So prayer or positive thinking creates less space for negative mental chatter. Prayer is used by many musicians to keep their hearts and minds clear of negative thoughts and experiences. I have seen many artists pray for a great show right before they go onstage.

USE THE POWER OF AFFIRMATIONS

I learned about "second thoughts" from an AA/Buddhist friend in Las Vegas. I share this with my patients who get stuck in negative or judgmental thought patterns. You rarely have control over your first or immediate thoughts and emotions related to a situation. "First thoughts" are usually a result of social conditioning, family programming, media, and society's norms. However, we can control our second thoughts and our reactions to them. This is the art of using affirmation and visualizations to reprogram our beliefs and silence our inner critic.

Start by taking an inventory of your typical negative "first thoughts": I'm unhappy, I'm poor, I'm fat, I'm undeserving, I'm stupid. For each negative first thought, invent a healthier second thought that you would prefer to believe instead, such as: I'm happy, I'm beautiful, I'm abundant, I'm thin, I'm worthy, I'm brilliant. When you find yourself mired in a first thought, replace it with your more positive mantra. In time, you'll reprogram your mind to focus on positive affirmations and your second thoughts will become your new reality.

FIND YOUR CREATIVITY

Creativity is one of the joys of being human. It adds color to a black-and-white world. It adds meaning and purpose. It gives us the ability to find solutions and is the way we celebrate our gifts and uniqueness in the world.

We're all creative by nature. It requires nothing more than the innate human qualities we were born with: openness, curiosity, passion, desire, inspiration, enthusiasm, and fearlessness in trying something new. It doesn't necessarily mean you're writing a book or dancing or singing. Perhaps you have a creative way of parenting or cooking. Or you may express your creativity in the way you dress or the way you decorate your house. Maybe it's the way you design a garden or nurture your relationships. Some of my business clients are the most creative people I've ever met. They're innovative in the way they build companies and manage employees and make products. Think about your life and what ways you love to express your uniqueness and gifts.

HARM REDUCTION TECHNIQUE: UNPLUG YOUR CREATIVITY

Do you watch more than ten hours of television per week? If so, trade some of that TV time for social activities, exercise, or creative pursuits. Too much mindless television limits your engagement with others and stifles your creativity.

"I see all these people staring at their phone, texting and typing. There are great opportunities out there for human connection. You can learn so much by having a physical conversation with another human being. This is something your phone can't teach you. Music is that conversation. It connects people. It is the universal language that everyone understands."

—MARK BATSON, PRODUCER,
ALICIA KEYS, DAVE MATTHEWS, EMINEM

If you're feeling blocked, stimulate your creativity by being open and curious, trying new adventures, taking on different projects at home or work, clearing your mind to create space for ideas, being more playful, experiencing joy, using your nondominant hand. It doesn't matter how inspired you feel in this moment: know that creativity cultivates more creativity. The more you practice, the more it stirs your inner fire and desire to create and be more of who you really are.

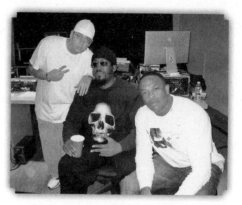

MARK BATSON WITH EMINEM AND DR. DRE
(COURTESY OF MARK BATSON)

NURTURE RELATIONSHIPS. LOVE IS THE DRUG!

Relationships are like the roots of a tree. They give you grounding and a sense of security. The deeper your roots the bigger the branches can be and the more fruitful and rewarding life can become. The rooting of relationships allows you to reach out for greater horizons and feel strength behind you. They offer you support in life. Cultivating strong personal relationships is essential for vitality and great health.

Whether you're cultivating new friendships or enhancing current relationships, there are a few things you can do to help them flourish:

- **GIVE TIME.** It's one of the best gifts you can offer another person. We rarely spend quality time just being with the ones we love. It is the most valuable gift and it is very affordable, too!

- **REALIZE THAT GIVING AND RECEIVING ARE THE SAME.** When you realize this, and that when you give you get just as much back, you open yourself up to deeper connections. Every exchange with another person is an opportunity to experience your version of a higher power in them.
- **LISTEN (FOR REAL).** Most people rarely feel truly heard or understood. Listen with compassion and without judgment. This opens you up to more intimacy.
- **SEEK TO UNDERSTAND.** Try to understand where others are coming from and imagine walking in their shoes before you judge them.
- **TAKE RESPONSIBILITY FOR YOURSELF ONLY.** When you take ownership of your actions and allow others to do the same you are freer to create the life you want for yourself.
- **INSPIRE OTHERS.** Don't try to change other people. We can only inspire them and motivate them by our own actions. If they don't follow your lead, let them be. They are their own change agents.
- **BE KIND, LOVING, COMPASSIONATE, AND FORGIVING.** This works especially well with people you have negative feelings toward. In other words, treat people the way you would like them to treat you. Offer forgiveness as a way to free yourself from negative resentments that are weighing you down.
- **KNOW YOUR BOUNDARIES.** And communicate them. It's healthier for everyone when you're honest with yourself and others.
- **LOSE THE BAGGAGE.** Past experiences are only baggage when you carry them with you into the present. Your personal history helped you learn and become the person you are now. But you don't have to let it define how you will be and what you will experience now. Be in the present moment with all of your relationships.

> "The secret to a healthy rock & roll marriage is trust, respect, an open mind, and never using the bathroom in front of each other."
> —PEARL ADAY, SINGER, MÖTLEY CRÜE, MEAT LOAF (LF)

FOR BETTER OR WORSE

I was invited to work on an artist at the opening concert for the Rock and Roll Hall of Fame. He wanted to get a massage to decompress from the stress of traveling. A few minutes into his treatment his ex-wife, who was also an artist performing that weekend, stormed into the room. She started in on him, asking him if he was planning to visit her mother while he was in town. He made every excuse under the sun as to why he could not go see his ex-mother-in-law. "I have interviews, I have rehearsal, I have sound check," blah, blah, blah.

She went into a fury: "You are such a jerk! You have not changed one bit. All you think about is yourself. It is such a small thing to ask. How could you do this to me, again?" She stormed out, apologizing to me.

After she left he called her names and said he was a fool to marry her, but he got some nice kids out of the deal. Even though they were acting hateful, I could tell they still loved each other. The massage continued on like a therapy session. I asked if he liked his mother-in-law. He said she was a great lady, so I suggested that he take an hour to go see her. This would make his ex-wife and mother-in-law happy and he would get a home-cooked meal. Eventually he came around to the idea and called his ex to say he would go. (I told him that the counseling was included in the price of the massage.) In doing so, he was relieved of his own guilt and animosity, and he made two people he cared about happy.

I was taken by the humanness of this interaction. These iconic stars were dealing with the same things that we all deal with in negotiating relationships. Somehow, onstage they seem elevated from the problems of ordinary people, but we are really all the same.

VISUALIZE YOUR DREAMS

Some people believe that you can manifest your dreams by visualizing, believing, and feeling them as if they've actually happened already. It's a technique used by many rockers before they go onstage—visualizing a successful performance—as well as elite-level athletes who visualize their winning performances while training. This isn't a new philosophy, but one that I've found to be common to a lot of my clients. They use it to overcome stage fright, play a new instrument, or conjure up a great performance.

Visualization accesses the power of your thoughts to make your wishes and desires a reality. You can use this practice by focusing on what you truly imagine for yourself. Where do you want to be? What does that look like, smell like, taste like? How do you feel in your body and mind? What do your relationships look like? How does your body perform? An easy place to start is with gratitude and giving thanks as if your dream has already come true. Thank you for this amazing new job, thank you for letting me pay off my bills, thank you for this loving relationship.

Practice this for a minute or two each morning and night and throughout the day to keep your vision alive and moving toward greater health. When you take your dreams out of the clouds and make them an adventure, they become your reality. Remember, this should be fun!

CONNECT TO A SPIRITUAL OR RELIGIOUS PRACTICE

Religion and spirituality are traditions and rituals that help us connect to divine energies. In their essence they add a deeper dimension to ordinary life and can provide us with a community and context for understanding. Learning about the religion and spiritual practice of my patients helps me to understand the lens through which they are approaching life and the beliefs that may affect their healing.

Religion and spirituality can be incorporated into your metaphor for healing. For example the detox may be used while one is practicing spiritual detox, such as Yom Kippur, Ramadan, fasting, confession, and the fourth and fifth steps of twelve-step programs. The common threads of spiritual practice and religions are the practice of surrender, devotion, forgiveness, prayer, sharing and connecting to others, kindness and compassion, and gratitude. All of these principles are part of a path to healing the body, mind, and spirit.

HIGHWAY TO HEAVEN

I was asked to work with a famous "death metal" band that I had never heard of before. I was nervous about what they would be like after seeing super-scary photos of them online. I had visions of animal sacrifices and satanic rituals backstage. They looked like an ominous bunch, but I was up for the adventure. I arrived with my equipment and my natural medicine road show and was escorted backstage. The first thing I saw was a cute little toddler racing around on a Big Wheel wearing a heavy metal T-shirt. His nanny was chasing him around the halls of the theater.

As usual, the lead singer gets his treatment first. While waiting for him, I noticed there was no alcohol in the back-stage beverage area. When he arrived, he was a soft-spoken guy and had the Serenity Prayer from AA posted on his dressing room mirror. Apparently, he was clean and sober. As the night unfolded, I learned that one of the guitarists was a born-again Christian. He wore a cross around his neck and kept a Bible in his dressing room. Another guitarist was into yoga and found an Indian guru to be his teacher. Each member had his own spiritual path.

They were one of the sweetest groups that I have ever met and one of the few who truly seem to get along. Yet each one was so different. They often teased each other about their spiritual leanings, but at the same time, they really respected each other. It was "unity in diversity" and it is true: you can't judge a book by its cover.

EMBRACE THERAPY

Smashing guitars and destroying hotel rooms isn't enough to re-solve anger and pent-up issues . . . even for rock stars. It's not very sociable or affordable, either. Therapy can be a healthy way to understand thought patterns that have led you to where you are in life and the experiences that cause anger, depression, pain, and trauma. It's also great for helping you get unstuck if you find yourself in a rut. A good therapist is simply facilitating healing and self-understanding to get you in a place of being in the moment without the baggage.

My clients incorporate psychotherapy styles that address the mind and spirit, such as creative arts therapy, transpersonal therapy, psychoanalysis, somatic therapies, and/or mind-body therapy. That said, therapy doesn't have to come from a couch session. Many find healing or new momentum through artistic expression or support from friends or even exercise. Others prefer coaching, which focuses more on the present moment and explores where you are at, where you would like to be, and the steps to move you there.

SOME KIND OF MONSTER

This 2004 award-winning documentary, filmed and produced by Joe Berlinger and Bruce Sinofsky, follows the legendary heavy metal band Metallica through the making of the 2003 album *St. Anger*. The movie is an intimate portrayal of the trials, tribulations, and triumphs that the band goes through as they work through their personal demons and relationship challenges. The band management, Q Prime, hires a performance coach who helps to facilitate dialogue between the members of Metallica as they navigate the stresses of addiction recovery, members quitting, interpersonal conflicts, creative blocks, and individual desires for more balance of band life and home life. It is a great example of how coaching and therapy can be used in relationships to heal wounds and move toward a common goal, which in this case was a great album!

REST AND RELAX YOUR MIND AND SPIRIT

Rest and relaxation are essential to being effective and present in body, mind, and spirit. We need time to completely relax and come out of the "fight or flight" mode and the stress of daily living in order to have high-quality attention and presence in our life. The following are ways we can rest and rejuvenate our body, mind, and spirit.

AROMATHERAPY

Aromatherapy practitioners use aromatic plant compounds, known as "essential oils," to harmonize emotional, physical, and spiritual imbalances. Essential oils are the immune system of the plant. The component that gives them their strong aroma also protects them from bacteria and viruses and other microbes. These oils will also do the same for you. They enhance your immune function and protect you from infections that will slow you down. Other benefits vary depending on the active constituents in the specific oil and plant, but in general they increase your well-being and happiness, decrease anxiety, balance or boost your energy, improve your immune system, and help you sleep more soundly.

There are four ways to use these fragrant oils: (1) diffuse 1–2 drops in the air with a diffuser; (2) inhale directly from a cloth or bottle; (3) add several drops to bathwater; or (4) apply 1–2 drops topically either directly under your nose or 3–5 drops to a carrier oil, like almond oil. Essential oils work because of their pharmacological effects on your physiology, and because of their olfactory effects on the limbic system of your brain. You can use them daily in a bath to help relax before bed, at the office for more energy, or in massage and body oils. I use them on rock stars during their backstage massages to enhance the benefits of their particular treatments as well as to get them energized or relaxed, depending on their specific need.

Channel your inner rock star with these oils:

- **BASIL** for burnout and exhaustion
- **EUCALYPTUS** for cough and sinuses
- **FRANKINCENSE** to channel creativity and connect spiritually
- **LAVENDER** for insomnia and anxiety
- **MYRRH** for throat health and self-expression
- **PATCHOULI** for the "dead heads"
- **PEPPERMINT** for inflammation and pain
- **ROSE** to enhance radiance and open the heart to love
- **ROSEMARY** for creativity, brain power, memory, and hair loss
- **TEA TREE OIL** for athlete's foot and fungal infections
- **THYME** for colds and chest infections
- **YLANG-YLANG** for depression

REIKI

Reiki, an energy-based healing art that originated in Japan, allows the universal life force to channel through a practitioner's hands to the client's body to harmonize energy. The Reiki practitioner has received an "attunement," which allows them to pass on the universal life force energy. This is a very subtle and soothing treatment and can be used for just about any ailment. I find it particularly helpful for supporting mind/body conditions such as anxiety, fatigue, grief, insomnia, depression, chronic illness, and stage fright. It brings the client into a balance of body and mind and restores the feelings of well-being that may have been lost due to chronic stress, trauma, or illness. Try it at least once. If you feel the benefits then talk to your Reiki practitioner about recommended frequency for your particular needs.

"There are things that I need on tour to help me stay connected. I take my dogs on tour with me, everywhere. As impossible as it sometimes is, having them with me is very healing. And nature is my game, even just visiting a zoo! Other things that have helped a bit on tour are Reiki, massage, some yoga, and this meditation I do: I touch my pulse and my chest and I breathe."

—CHAN MARSHALL, SINGER, SONGWRITER, CAT POWER

SLEEP

Sleep is one of the most important factors in a healthy RxStar lifestyle. We know from research that people need about seven to nine hours of sleep each night, with established bedtimes and wake times. That's a fantasy for most of us. Sleep is often the first thing that gets sacrificed when life gets overbooked, whether for work or play. It's also one of the most difficult areas to regulate, but critical because the quality of your sleep profoundly affects the quality of your waking life and health. When you compromise the number of hours your body needs, you miss out on the four stages of sleep: transition to sleep, light sleep, deep sleep, and REM sleep. While you're resting, your body keeps working. Deep quality sleep and REM sleep allows your body to repair, boosts immunity function, regenerates organs and cells, combats aging, repairs muscles and tissues, prevents disease, elevates your mood, helps with weight loss, strengthens memory, and increases neurotransmitters such as serotonin and dopamine.

Your internal twenty-four-hour sleep-wake cycle, aka your biological clock or circadian rhythm, is regulated by the brain's response to waking hours and light and dark periods. At night, your body produces melatonin, a hormone necessary for sleep. During the day, sunlight triggers the brain to inhibit melatonin production, making you feel awake and alert.

Many factors disrupt the sleep/wake cycle and affect the quality of sleep, such as night-shift work, late-night concerts and parties, traveling across time zones, irregular sleeping patterns, artificial light, stress, and nutritional factors. Melatonin production can also be thrown off if you don't get enough sunlight exposure during the day and have exposure to artificial light at night, especially light from electronic devices, including TVs, computers, tablets, and mobile phones.

"I have a mental ritual I use to help me go to sleep. It is a visualization exercise in which I focus on each area of my body and allow it to relax. The throat is one of the main areas you must relax before you go to sleep. If you are having trouble sleeping, then the full-body relaxation will expedite it faster."
—MIKE MILLS, SONGWRITER, BASSIST, AND KEYBOARDIST, R.E.M.

15 WAYS TO IMPROVE YOUR SLEEP QUALITY

At minimum, I recommend 7 hours of sleep per night. For maintenance, aim for 8–10 hours per night, and for repair and healing, shoot for 10–12 hours. Remember, quality is just as important as quantity.

1. Abstain from coffee, alcohol, sugar, or nicotine before bed for three hours.
2. Add daily melatonin supplements—3 mg before bed is ideal.
3. Avoid big meals at night.
4. Eat more protein in the evening and fewer carbs or sugar.
5. Drink herbal teas for relaxation: chamomile, passionflower, oats, skullcap.
6. Increase sunlight exposure during the day to boost melatonin.
7. Make your bedroom a "Keith Richards Room," that is, very dark with no light, for those who like to sleep all day and party all night.
8. Sleep at the same time daily.
9. Sleep when it is dark and stay awake when it is light if you can.
10. Take calcium, magnesium, and vitamin D at night (see bottles for dosage).
11. Turn off the TV, cell phones, and computers one hour before bed.
12. Use a firm mattress with a soft top.
13. Use calming techniques one hour before bed: read, meditate, stretch, have sex, or be in nature (or all of the above).

14. Use light boxes in winter or if you are a night worker or live in a dark area.
15. Wake at the same time daily.

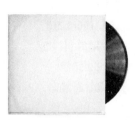

BONUS TRACKS

"I quit all the drugs and alcohol over twenty years back, and that was the biggest game changer in my life. From there flowed my workouts, diets, massages, and other healthy lifestyle regimens. It has also given a thirst to my soul to be fed as well. If I hit the gym, my body is fit; when I nourish the soul, my spirit stays fit. I'm open to all spiritual ideas and I'm a regular church attendee, read the Bible, and do my daily devotions as well. More important, I find it best to carry out those things in all my daily activities of trying to be helpful and courteous to others in my life. In the world of the spirit, giving it away to keep it is the key. So, whether on tour or at home, I try to contribute to life, rather than just be a consumer."

—DAVE ELLEFSON, BASSIST, MEGADETH

"If you have already soothed your mind and washed your soul through meditation or prayer, you are better equipped to deal with loved ones. My wife was deep into it, and it was natural to follow her lead. It has been good for our relationship. Stopping and being calm and taking a moment to do eye meditations—just look at each other in the eyes . . . it is never a bad thing to do."

—KIRK DOUGLAS, GUITARIST, **THE ROOTS**

"I do this thing called 'emotional freedom tapping technique.' I tap acupuncture points and say positive mantras to myself. There are different sorts of voodoo rituals to get you into the mode of playing in front of people. One of the most common is drugs and alcohol. But you can do this in a healthy way, too: Yoga, EFT, mantra, and meditation are all things that work for that."

—**JOSEPH ARTHUR,** SINGER, SONGWRITER, GUITARIST

"I always pray before I go onstage. I'm not dogmatically religious, but I check in. I see God as someone quite loving. I will pray that the music somehow will reach somebody, on some level, regardless of what it is. I would also say that I find music is prayer."

—PAUL CANTELON, FILM SCORE COMPOSER, PIANIST, ACCORDIONIST, VIOLINIST, **WILD COLONIALS**

"We were all trained in the New York school of never staying frozen. Creativity is not a luxury. You wake up in the morning, go to an office or studio or your instrument and be creative. It's a profession. You don't smoke pot and wait for the muse. You practice creativity as a muscle."

—ORI KAPLAN, SAXOPHONIST, **BALKAN BEAT BOX**

"I go everywhere with my Brain Machine. It is a light and sound device that works on synchronizing the alpha, beta, theta, and delta rhythms. Deepak Chopra has one called the Dream Weaver. You can program it for creativity, to pacify yourself, or to energize yourself. I do it on trains, planes, and anywhere I am waiting a long time. They haven't locked me away yet!"

—MICK ROCK, ROCK & ROLL PHOTOGRAPHER

"I love to go fishing. I started fishing when I was seven years old. It was a way for me to spend time with my father. When I am fishing, there is no mind on the music or the problems. I just lay back and listen to the water, the bees, the mosquitoes, and the birds. It gives me peace."

—SHARON JONES, SINGER,
SHARON JONES & THE DAP-KINGS

"I really like essential oils, aromatherapy, acupuncture, and massage. All these things are very important for destressing the body and mind. They help me to focus and help my muscles to withstand what I put them through! I use lavender oil to help me to relax and eventually sleep."

—MÁIRÉAD NESBITT, FIDDLER AND VIOLINIST,
CELTIC WOMAN

"I found a bit of strength and I thought, 'Well, you know I refuse to even say the word (cancer).' Even now I never said the word (cancer). I did do both, chemo and radiation. I just put it in my head like I was going to the spa. I would go there, and obviously Sloan-Kettering is like a seven-star hotel, it's so beautiful. You would have the lounge and the fucking chair that looked like British Airways first class. I'd take my iPod, grab my lipstick, and

I'd be all dolled up. When I'd come out, I would go and spend $600 on a pair of shoes, a wallet, or a bag. The shock of spending $600 took away any kind of shock about just having poison put in my body."

—ANGELA MCCLUSKEY, SINGER, SONGWRITER,
TELEPOP, WILD COLONIALS

"Sleep's a precious thing. I get insomnia from exhaustion. I'll get to the point where I'm so exhausted on a tour that my mind's not computing things right. I might feel a weird pain and instead of just thinking that I slept on it wrong, I think that I'm having a heart attack or something. It makes you have an overactive imagination, and then the next thing you know, you are like fucking Woody Allen."

—CONOR OBERST, SINGER, SONGWRITER, GUITARIST,
BRIGHT EYES, LOS DESAPARECIDOS

"I have been interested in Eastern and Native American philosophy since I was a kid. I don't consider Eastern philosophy to be exotic or esoteric or objectify or analyze my processes; I just remain open to new insights and information that can add to a broader awareness and deeper insights."

—IAN ASTBURY, **THE CULT**

"After I got sober, what turned into a really interesting perspective on a city I was visiting was going to the local gym. It's a really neat way to mix with local people. That, coupled with bike riding, gives you a geographic feel for the city. Honestly, I don't even like riding in itself, it's not my thing. The only reason I do the AIDS Ride Life cycle (the yearly charity bike ride from San Francisco to LA) is that I like to make money for the cause. It's a really fun, special trip, a really crazy, wonderful experience. It's 550 miles in total; it takes a week, and six nights in a tent."

—RODDY BOTTUM, KEYBOARDIST, **FAITH NO MORE**

CHAPTER 10

STAGE FIVE: SOCIALIZE AND CELEBRATE GOOD TIMES!

Being healthy doesn't mean being boring! Socializing is a key part of vibrant health. Countless studies have shown that all the perks of leisure time, from laughter to friendships to fun activities, add to our happiness, vitality, and longevity.

The key to being a healthy social butterfly is making sure you adhere to the 90/10 Rule. Does that mean you only get to enjoy life 10 percent of the time, while 90 percent is zero fun? Absolutely not! It simply means that in the midst of following what brings you joy, you remember to stay healthy *most* of the time. You implement the Harm Reduction Techniques, follow the diet guidelines when you eat out (when you can), and pay attention to how your body feels. If you begin losing energy, getting sick, or experiencing any of the many symptoms of living at 80-20 or 70-30, it's time to look at where you're slipping.

I'm realistic. I know that living a work-hard, play-hard life means occasionally overindulging in cocktails or junk food, sneaking a cigarette here or there, or skimping on sleep to hang out with friends. That's why I designed this chapter to give you all the tools you need to maximize your health without sacrificing your fun. You'll learn the best ways to navigate social situations so you don't have to miss the party to stay healthy.

RxSTAR RESTAURANT GUIDE

Eating at restaurants, parties, or events can be part of the 90 percent or the 10 percent, depending on the choice of food or establishment. The best options are typically those that serve healthy organic options, farm-to-table, or local cuisine. If you're a less adventurous eater, good health can be an excellent motivator for experimenting with and learning the experience of cultures and cuisine as well as celebrating with friends and family in a new way.

> "If you are unhappy and unfulfilled and looking for food to be a way to make yourself fulfilled, then you are going to sit there and eat the whole plate and more! And you are going to feel like shit afterward. It's like you don't eat all the candy in the candy store. Don't be greedy. Don't be gluttonous. Satisfy yourself and do it in a way that is better for you and that works."
>
> —RUSSELL SIMINS, DRUMMER,
> **JON SPENCER BLUES EXPLOSION**

Harm Reduction Techniques for Eating Out:

Restaurants, airports, office cafeterias, and house parties aren't always a mecca of good nutrition. Fortunately, there are ways to limit their negative impact. Try these guidelines:

- **LOOK FOR RESTAURANTS** that offer vegetarian or locally grown ingredients, or choose family-run ethnic spots.
- **IF ORGANIC ISN'T ON THE MENU,** order entrees made with lamb, wild-caught fish, goat or sheep dairy, or vegetables.
- **LIMIT YOURSELF** to 1 cup of cooked rice, no matter what type of fare or restaurant.
- **FOR REDUCED OR NO GLUTEN,** look for Thai, Vietnamese, Chinese, Indian, Mexican/South American, or Middle Eastern (limit the bread) meals.
- **CHOOSE HEALTHIER FAST-FOOD OPTIONS,** such as vegetable burritos, fish tacos, mushroom quesadillas, falafel sandwiches/platters, lamb gyros, shish kebabs, wraps, soups, yogurt with toppings, or salads with vegetables and protein.
- **AT ASIAN ESTABLISHMENTS,** ask for no MSG, avoid fried items, and get dishes loaded with veggies (tempura doesn't count!).
- **AT THE MEXICAN CANTINA,** switch from refried to black beans, avoid sour cream, choose fish over chicken or beef, add veggies to burritos and tacos, and pass on the corn chips or have only a few (I know, yeah, right!) unless they're blue corn.
- **IN ITALIAN PLACES,** start with the vegetable antipasti, go gluten-free with risotto or entrees with veggies and meat or fish, or choose low-gluten items like gnocchi or eggplant parmigiana.

- **AT BURGER JOINTS**, skip the bun (or use lettuce, a tortilla, or pita instead), bag the fries for a salad, and choose organic meats or wild game if possible.
- **OPT FOR MY FAVORITE ONE-BITE WONDER—SUSHI.** It's perfect for detox and post-detox diets because: (1) ginger stimulates digestive enzymes; (2) rice protects the GALT; (3) seaweed pulls out mercury; (4) wasabi kills parasites; and (5) wild fish contains omega-3s and protein. Don't forget to chase your sushi roll with a cup of green tea for an antioxidant boost.
- **WHEN EATING GREEK, TURKISH, OR LEBANESE,** load up on healthy appetizers—think olives, olive oil, hummus, falafel, baba ghanoush, yogurt dips, vegetables stuffed with nuts or rice, wild fish, or salads like tabouli, fattoush, or Greek.
- **SWITCH SODA** for coconut water, glass-bottled iced tea or water, spritzers with soda water and juice, or fruit juices diluted in water at a 1:3 ratio.
- **CHOOSE BIODYNAMIC OR ORGANIC WINES** to avoid the pesticides. Or have Italian, Spanish, or French wines, which are usually lower in pesticides, if organic is not an option.
- **IF IT'S IMPOSSIBLE TO NIX THE BREAD BASKET,** eat the yummy crust only, and with a little olive oil.

PARTY HEALTHY

While it's well known that alcohol can be rough on the liver, what's less known is that certain substances impact how the organ metabolizes spirits. For example, grapefruit contains naringenin, which slows the detox of alcohol from the liver; therefore the alcohol stays in your blood longer.

The formula is simple: Grapefruit + Spirits = Bigger Buzz

The upside is that when you mix grapefruit juice with alcohol, you need to drink half as much to get the same high. This is a very effective Harm Reduction Technique I use with rock stars to decrease their alcohol intake if they are not ready to cut out alcohol completely. They have a drink mixed with a little grapefruit juice and they drink less. The downside is that if you add grapefruit juice to your cocktails, but still drink heavily, you'll most likely get very drunk! Consider yourself warned!

HARM REDUCTION TECHNIQUE: JUICY FRUIT

Fruit juice counts as several servings of fruit and it's metabolized as food. Unfortunately, too much fruit juice can suppress immune function, just like sugar does. If you want a juice fix, drink only organic fruit juices and dilute them with one-third juice and two-thirds filtered water.

Other ingredients that slow the detox of alcohol from the liver:

- CLOVE
- DRUGS—ANTIHISTAMINES, BENZODIAZEPINES, ANTACIDS, SSRIs, SOME ANTIBIOTICS AND ANTIFUNGALS
- KAVA KAVA
- SAINT-JOHN'S-WORT
- TURMERIC

Just as there are substances that increase the effects of alcohol on your liver, others protect the organ from the wear and tear of happy hour.

Try the following foods and supplements (per bottle dosage instructions) on nights you drink:

ANTIOXIDANTS AND BIOFLAVONOIDS: also found in fruits (especially lemon and lime), dark-skinned berries, vegetables, and green tea

GLUTATHIONE-CYSTEINE, GLUTAMINE, GLYCINE: amino acids that support liver detoxification

METHIONINE: an amino acid also found in eggs, fish, Brazil nuts, and seeds

MILK THISTLE: an herb long known to protect the liver, available in capsules and teas

MSM: a sulfur also found in eggs, onions, garlic, and cruciferous vegetables like kale, broccoli, cauliflower, and cabbage

VITAMIN B: also found in legumes, greens, nuts, meat, and fish

VITAMIN C: also found in citrus fruits and vegetables

VITAMIN E: also found in nuts, seeds, and whole grains

Whether you're partaking in a monthlong detox, a recovery program, or simply a night off from cocktailing, social situations like bars and parties can be challenging. Well-meaning friends, family, coworkers, and party hosts often don't take "no thank you" for an answer. Dodging the inevitable questioning or prodding is easier when you have a drink in hand. Mentally, it can help you feel more "celebratory" and less awkward in social situations.

Try these non-alcoholic bar options:

ARNOLD PALMER: a 50-50 split of iced tea and lemonade

BITTERS AND SODA OR TONIC

BROWN PELICAN: apple cider and ginger beer

CRANBERRY JUICE AND LIME

GUNNER: ginger beer, ginger ale, Angostura bitters, and a splash of lime cordial

HENRY: orange juice and lemonade

JEFFERSON: iced tea and orange juice

LEMON, LIME, & BITTERS (LLB): lemonade, lime juice, and bitters

MICHELANGELO: orange juice and tonic water

NON-ALCOHOLIC BEERS: O'Doul's, Kaliber, Buckler, Sharp's, Coors NA, or Busch NA

REBECCA: pineapple juice, cranberry juice, and soda water

ROCK SHANDY: soda water, lemonade, and a dash of Angostura bitters

SAFE SEX ON THE BEACH: cranberry juice, grapefruit juice, and peach nectar

SPARKLING GRAPE JUICE

VIRGIN MARY: a Bloody Mary without the vodka

RxSTAR REMEDY HANGOVER CURES

Sometimes the day after drinking can make you never want to drink again. The good news is that there are healthier "cures" for the morning after than a greasy cheeseburger and fries. Try my Backstage Alternatives to replenish much-needed vitamins, minerals, and fluids:

DETOX: A good place to start is the detox shake. Using it as part of the detox leads to a cleaner liver, but it can also be used on the morning after to help you replenish lost vitamins and bounce back. Also, the more hydrated you are, the more your symptoms will ease. Replenish with electrolyte replacements like coconut water and vegetable bouillon along with 8–10 glasses of water to flush toxins.

NOURISH AND HYDRATE: Pass on the leftover pizza and eat easy-to-digest foods like oatmeal, rice, and soup.

SUPPLEMENT: B-complex, Emergen-C (1–2 packets daily), and vitamin C (1,000 mg) to replenish your vitamin levels. Add herbal remedies to support your liver, like dandelion tea (1–2 cups) or milk thistle (per bottle instructions).

TREAT: Get at least 8–10 hours of sleep. A sauna, steam, or exercise will help you sweat out the toxins. And if you can get to your acupuncturist, ask for add-on acupuncture points: ST 36, LI 4, ST 44, LV3, PC 6.

RxSTAR HEALTHY TRAVEL TIPS

Whether you're traveling for work, play, or rejuvenation, there are tricks for keeping your time on the road healthy.

Travel for Work/Touring

For many rock stars and business travelers, being on the road is an extension of daily life and where 60–80 percent of their time is spent. *This is their life.* When you're home only 20 percent of your life, you can't just say, "I'm going to get healthy when I'm done working." You must make your routine the same on the road as it is at home. You will need to have a system in place before you leave that allows you to be healthy without sacrificing your lifestyle; otherwise it's nearly impossible to achieve or maintain vitality. You have to figure out how to build your health routine into travel mode because this is the life you created.

Then change your consciousness about it—learn to love and enjoy it. After all, it's giving you abundance and experiences so be sure to appreciate it and make the best of it.

People Get Ready

When you're constantly on the go, it's much more difficult to stick to the 90-10 Rule by winging it. Instead, build your healthy lifestyle on the road. Sure, you're probably not traveling on private jets or tour buses outfitted like rolling apartments, but you can make travel seamless and healthy so that transitioning from the road to home is an easy adjustment.

Use this checklist to streamline the process from the beginning:

- ✔ Separate supplies for home and travel to make it easy, convenient, and instantly packable.
- ✔ Keep a toiletries bag packed with nontoxic beauty and grooming supplies.
- ✔ Keep luggage ready to go and stocked with your different regimens—in fact, when I prepare for a trip, all I do is add clothes to my suitcase.
- ✔ Stock an arsenal of healthy snacks to have on hand for hotels, buses, and planes.
- ✔ Keep self-help and spiritual books packed or downloaded.

- ✔ Download online workouts or bring CDs, plus a tablet, phone, or computer.
- ✔ Pack your traveler's first-aid kit.
- ✔ Pack the RxStar Detox Shake supplies and supplements.
- ✔ Bring personal items that will make every hotel room feel like it's your own room, such as pictures, candles, and incense.
- ✔ Connect to loved ones and friends before you leave and stay connected while you're away.
- ✔ Be in the moment and grateful so that even the travel prep becomes enjoyable.

Travel for Pleasure (Vacation)

Everyone needs a break in routine to relax, rejuvenate, and recharge the body, mind, and spirit, whether that means a beach holiday, yoga retreat, or hiking trip. Some of us rejuvenate through doing absolutely nothing. Others need some real activity that allows them to let off steam and release tension.

Choose a vacation that balances what you are lacking in your daily life. For instance, if you are working seventy-hour weeks doing physical activity and burning out, then ten days of sleep, massage, and beach lounging may be perfect for you. However, if your job is sedentary and mentally draining, an active vacation with loads of hiking, biking, and yoga may be just what the doctor ordered. Regardless of how you choose to spend your downtime, a few guidelines can help you maximize your trip:

- CATCH UP ON SLEEP AND EXERCISE.
- CHECK EMAILS AND INTERNET ONLY ONCE PER DAY.

- LET YOUR MIND BE FREE FROM THE CONSTANT BARRAGE OF INFORMATION AND ENJOY THE SPACE TO LET YOUR MIND WANDER. THIS ENHANCES CREATIVITY AND LETS YOUR BRAIN CELLS REST.
- TRY TO PICK AN ACTIVITY OR AREA THAT ALLOWS YOU TO EAT HEALTHY.
- UNPLUG FROM CONSTANT ELECTRONIC STIMULATION.
- USE CELL PHONES ONLY FOR EMERGENCIES.

Travel for Adventure, Exploration, or Experience

This is my favorite form of travel and where I find I'm the most open, aware, and fully present. When you're in a new country or environment or culture, you're completely immersed in the moment and because everything is so new, you're often always on your toes and aware of what's happening around you. It allows you to be fully present and experience a completely new lens on the world and its inhabitants. It's excellent for sharing cultures and healing intolerance and prejudices. And it can remind you that there is more going on in life than the mundane everyday issues that cause stress and anxiety and anger.

Many artists often love this type of travel—although it's challenging with their schedules—because it sparks creativity and opens awareness to new ideas or ways of seeing the world. It clears your mind and exposes you to different perspectives. Others, like Bono, travel to places like Africa to meet the people and make a difference in their lives. Bono gathers information and learns about a culture so he can make an impact on the world.

Maximize this travel by:
✔ Dining at local restaurants

- ✔ Learning phrases in the native tongue, like hello, good-bye, thank you, how are you?
- ✔ Leaving a small footprint environmentally and socially
- ✔ Losing expectations about having the same things you have at home
- ✔ Respecting local dress and customs
- ✔ Sharing your culture with them
- ✔ Speaking to the locals and learning about their culture

RxSTAR REMEDY HEALTHY OFFICE TIPS

The office is where most of us spend more than 50 percent of our lives; therefore it's important to set up the environment to be healthy, comfortable, and a happy place to be. The idea is to create a space that you enjoy, not dread, one that makes you more productive and successful. To spend the majority of your office hours wishing you were somewhere else is not a waste of time; it's a waste of your life.

Mike D's Smoothie Recipe

1 fresh banana
1 tbsp almond butter
1 tbsp cacao
1 tbsp maca powder
protein or green powder of choice
pitted dates to taste
1 pint water

> "Blend that shit up in a Vitamix and drink it.
> Excellent for an afternoon or an energy boost."
>
> —MIKE D (DIAMOND), RAPPER, SONGWRITER, DRUMMER, AND PRODUCER,
> ## BEASTIE BOYS

> "Since discovering I have fibromyalgia, my diet has gotten better both on tour and off. In general, it's hard when you travel and it takes extra effort to eat clean. The best way is to keep a cooler in the car and hit grocery stores along the way, rather than try to eat healthy at a restaurant."
>
> —HOLLY MIRANDA, SINGER, SONGWRITER-MUSICIAN

Create Your Own Space

Step one is to style your space so that it reflects your character, creativity, and ambience. That might mean photos, inspirational mantras, plants, colors, designs, and items from home. The point is not to make this your home away from home, but rather to keep you inspired, empowered, energetic, and passionate. If you can't make work a happy experience, it will negatively impact your health.

There are a number of ways to detoxify and energize you and your space:

- ✔ Be grateful for a job that brings you security and money.
- ✔ Bring in a plant to oxygenate the air.
- ✔ Drink filtered water out of glass, ceramic, or stainless steel.
- ✔ Have an ergonomics evaluation of your

workspace to reduce risk of neck and back problems, carpal tunnel syndrome, and eye strain.

- ✔ Incorporate desk stretches and yoga poses.
- ✔ Keep two essential oils at your desk—energizing rosemary and calming lavender.
- ✔ Learn local healthy restaurants for delivery, takeout, and dining in.
- ✔ Stock up on healthy snacks each week or month: nuts, dried fruit, and high-quality protein bars.
- ✔ Take fresh air breaks and walk during lunch or downtime.
- ✔ Use a chair with good back support.
- ✔ Walk around the office when you can—it's a great excuse to connect with coworkers in person and build relationships.

Unplugged: Harm Reduction Techniques for the Office

The following recommendations will help to protect you from the excesses of radiation that come from all the electronic devices that you use or surround you:

- BATHE IN EPSOM SALTS WEEKLY.
- EAT DARK GREEN FOODS, SEAWEED, AND WILD-CAUGHT SEAFOOD TO INCREASE CHLOROPHYLL AND IODINE, WHICH PROTECT US FROM RADIATION EXPOSURE AND THYROID PROBLEMS.
- PLACE A BAG OF EPSOM SALTS NEXT TO THE COMPUTER TO DRAW RADIATION AWAY FROM YOU.

- SEASON FOOD WITH SEA SALT CONTAINING IODINE.
- SWIM IN THE OCEAN, A NATURAL RADIATION DETOXIFIER, WHEN POSSIBLE.
- USE RADIATION SCREENS.
- USE COMPUTERS INSTEAD OF LAPTOPS; PLACE THEM TWO FEET FROM YOU.

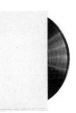

BONUS TRACKS

"I love kava kava. It's a root from Polynesia that is very calming. I was almost thrown out of City Winery by a bouncer who thought I was, like, dosing myself up. He was like, 'You can't do that here!' And I was like, 'It's from Whole Foods!' I was delighted that I looked so decadent. The best way is to mix it with very good bitters. Bitters and kava in sparkling water, and you feel like Iggy Pop without the lifestyle. I just do it as a total prop. But then everything is a prop in our lives."

—PAUL CANTELON, FILM SCORE COMPOSER, PIANIST, ACCORDIONIST, VIOLINIST, **WILD COLONIALS**

"I request on my rider that at each show I have a nice assortment of all kinds of berries. I love berries. I recently discovered Perky Jerky. It's a great snack. It contains guarana, a berry found in the Amazon that's in a lot of energy drinks."

—ORIANTHI, GUITARIST, **ALICE COOPER**

"Knowing wine and enjoying it have influenced my worldview by often being the entrance point for my personal discovery of world culture. The jump-starting, so to speak, of research about a particular place in the world, the wine, the food, the art, politics, language, and history. This, in turn, has influenced my music and writing."

—GEOFF TATE, SINGER, QUEENSRŸCHE

"I made a discovery of what every traveling person should have. I call it 'the Snake.' Ditch the crappy round-the-neck travel pillow. They got nothing on the Snake, which inflates and wraps around you, allowing fully upright supported sleep. It is made by Travel Rest. . . . If you have trouble resting while in transit, this will hook you up!"

—JORDAN MCLEAN, TRUMPETER,
ANTIBALAS, FIRE OF SPACE

"I started not eating any wheat or gluten. I encourage it even if you're not wheat intolerant, because it focuses your mind on eating other things that are healthier: "Hey, I can't have all those beers. What else can I have instead?" I'll have tequila. It's gluten free. It's fewer calories. And you don't chug it."

—SAUL SIMON MACWILLIAMS, KEYBOARDIST,
INGRID MICHAELSON

"I've realized you have to accept that there will some discomfort and inconvenience on the road, so you can either suck it up or you can go home. For me, going home isn't an option. I'm not going to chuck it over this. I deal with things now in a different way. I'm a realist."

—DEL STRIBLING, AKA "BINKY GRAPHITE," GUITARIST,
SHARON JONES & THE DAP-KINGS

CHARLEY DRAYTON'S ESSENTIAL
FIRST-AID KIT

Water with lemon every day
Ester C for the immune system
Probiotics
Digestive enzymes
Multivitamin
Primal Defense
Goldenseal
Natural cough syrup
Bio freeze for muscle pain

—CHARLEY DRAYTON, DRUMMER, BASSIST, AND PRODUCER,
FIONA APPLE, NEIL YOUNG, AND KEITH RICHARDS

"The most integral part of happy traveling is to stay positive, be patient, and have a sense of humor. Complaining is not going to make the situation better. We were traveling in Spain, and some of the guys were complaining about how long it takes for everything to happen there. Last time I checked in Spain, they have been moving slow for hundreds of years! So enjoy the culture of the country when you are there and try to adapt to it. Don't compare it to your life back home."

–KRAIG JARRET JOHNSON, GUITARIST, KEYBOARDS,
SINGER, SONGWRITER, ## RUN WESTY RUN, THE JAYHAWKS,
GOLDEN SMOG, JOSEPH ARTHUR

"I hardly ever drink anymore. For me, bottom line was I just couldn't take the hangovers anymore. I still love to drink; I just choose not to be hungover. Can't deal with it. It's a combination of the agony, the pain of the hangover, and the lost time. The idea of losing a day because I decided to get drunk just doesn't balance for me anymore."

—SCOTT IAN, GUITARIST, **ANTHRAX**

PART FOUR

HEAL, RESTORE, AND RECOVER

CHAPTER 11

THE CURES: ALTERNATIVE REMEDIES FOR ROCK STARS LIKE YOU

Congratulations! You've made it through the RxStar Remedy program. Even though you may have completed the RxStar Remedy Detox and are following the 90/10 Rules for food, fitness, and life, you may occasionally experience some of the side effects of living a full-on demanding lifestyle. After all, you're human!

In this section we'll look at alternative and holistic treatments I recommend for the most common issues I treat in my practice in-house and on tour, from fatigue to PMS to heartburn. These remedies include everything from nutrient-rich foods that alleviate particular symptoms to specific lifestyle changes that promote healing, to supplements and herbs that target certain issues or conditions. When used together, you'll be able to customize a treatment plan based on who you are and how you live. Like a RxStar!

As always, please consult your doctor or health practitioner before beginning any treatments, supplements, or medications.

1. ACNE

Acne is one of the most common skin conditions I treat and can be caused by a variety of factors, such as hormone imbalances, blood sugar imbalances, bacteria or skin infections, stress, and toxins. Acne can be one of the side effects of living life like a rock star. Because the skin is an organ of detoxification, it's not surprising that when your body is toxic and out of balance, your skin will let you know. Try my Backstage Alternatives to reduce redness, inflammation, breakouts, and other skin issues.

DETOX. The RxStar Detox eases symptoms and prevents further breakouts.

NOURISH AND HYDRATE. Eat foods that clear skin and prevent recurrence like dark leafy greens, yellow veggies for vitamin A, and garlic and onion for antibiotic power. Eliminate all white sugar, white flour, hydrogenated fats, cow's milk, alcohol, and soft drinks. Be sure to drink 8–10 glasses of water daily to flush toxins and keep cells functioning optimally.

SUPPLEMENT. If you're not already taking a food-based multivitamin and mineral supplement, add one daily plus: flaxseed oil (1 tablespoon daily); a probiotic supplement with *Lactobacillus acidophilus* (daily, per bottle instructions); and vitamins A (25,000 IU daily), E (400 IU daily), and D$_3$ (1,000 IU daily).

TREAT. There are many alternative treatments that help clear and prevent acne, including: weekly acupuncture facials; monthly organic cleaning facials; tea tree oil, a natural antibiotic, applied directly on acne; and argan oil, used a.m. and p.m. as a moisturizer, antibacterial agent, and anti-inflammatory (my favorite brand is Moroccan Elixir Ageless Face Oil, because it contains added essential oils to combat aging).

I ALSO RECOMMEND: cleansing and toning morning and night using an organic and natural product without petrochemicals; exercising 15–20 minutes daily to regulate hormones and expel dirt from pores when you sweat; and meditating 10–15 minutes per day minimum to relieve stress and balance hormones.

2. ALLERGIES (HAY FEVER)

Environmental allergies usually rear their head in spring and fall. And while you may want to blame mom or dad for your hereditary predisposition to the condition, it may also be a result of a weakened immune system or compromised adrenal function. Symptoms include: a runny nose, sinusitis, sneezing, itching eyes, fatigue, brain fog, sore throat, and headaches. Try my Backstage Alternatives for boosting your immunity and combating histamines:

DETOX. The RxStar Detox Shake boosts immunity, giving your body better fighting power against allergens. Follow it with my RxStar Immune Shake as a maintenance plan for allergies.

RxSTAR IMMUNE SHAKE
. . . .

I designed this immunity booster to deal with the many stresses and conditions that are common side effects of rock star lifestyles. Use it as a meal replacement for breakfast when cold and flu season are near or when you are feeling your immune system is challenged, and follow RxStar food recommendations for eating clean, whole foods.

Many clients use my RxStar Immune Shake, which you can re-create at home using the following nutritional combinations:

Pure whey (protein), 15 or more grams protein—2 scoops
Green food powder—1 scoop
Intestinal repair powder—2 teaspoons
Probiotic powder—½ teaspoon
Arctic cod liver oil or organic flaxseed oil—1 tablespoon

Mix the above ingredients into 12–16 ounces of purified water. You may add ½ cup of frozen organic fruit (you can add more, but watch the calories). Optional: add ½ cup yogurt or rice, almond, or soy milk. Note: Keep ingredients refrigerated. Consume in no less than 30 minutes—this is a meal, not a shot!

NOURISH AND HYDRATE. Eat citrus fruits and dark-skinned berries for vitamin C, along with red, yellow, and orange veggies for vitamin C and vitamin A. Add 1 teaspoon daily of local organic honey, a natural allergy fighter. Finally, eliminate all sugar, soft drinks, artificial sweeteners, wheat/gluten, and dairy products, which are common allergens and can increase inflammation. Round out the diet with 8–10 glasses of water daily.

SUPPLEMENT. Fight inflammation and allergens while boosting your immunity with: vitamin C (1,000 mg per day); food-based antioxidant formulas (daily, per bottle instructions); bioflavonoid formulas that include quercetin, rutin, and hesperidin (daily, per bottle instructions); proteolytic enzymes formulas with bromelain (daily, per bottle instructions); flaxseed oil (1 tablespoon daily); and a probiotic (daily, per bottle instructions). I recommend my clients with allergies also supplement with herbs like butterbur, elderberry, licorice root, and nettles.

TREAT. Add acupuncture and cranial sacral therapy weekly as well as daily use of a Neti pot or other forms of nasal irrigation to clean nasal passages.

3. ANXIETY

You can't expect to push yourself to the limit without feeling a little anxiety. After all, it's a common response to nervousness and stress. Symptoms include: mind racing, obsessive thoughts, worry, fear, avoidance of social situations, racing heart, shortness of breath, and trouble sleeping. The good news is that the remedies are surprisingly easy and effective.

Try my Backstage Alternatives to ease stress and improve your mood:

DETOX. The detox balances hormones and strengthens your body so you're better able to handle and lessen anxiety.

NOURISH. After detoxing, add to your diet foods that are rich in: vitamin B (tuna, turkey, beef); magnesium (beans and leafy greens); a natural sedative (oatmeal); and good-quality protein, eaten 3–4 times daily. Avoid sugar, alcohol, caffeine, nicotine, and sodas, which can cause mood fluctuations.

SUPPLEMENT. I recommend several supplements that can ease your stress and improve your mood, including: 5-HTP (50 mg daily); B-complex formula (daily, per bottle instructions); flax-seed oil (1 tablespoon daily); magnesium glycinate (300–400 mg daily with food); Rescue Remedy (5 drops, 3 times daily); and theanine (100 mg daily). Herbs are very effective as well: kava kava, passionflower, skullcap, and wild oats. Lavender essential oil is also very calming.

TREAT. Weekly acupuncture and massage treatments work wonders on stress levels. Add a daily meditation practice (15 minutes, minimum), along with walking or yoga 15 minutes per day at the very least to increase endorphins, circulation, and energy flow. If possible, get 8 hours of sleep per night and during the day, stay mindful. Being conscious of the present moment prevents you from worrying about the future or obsessing over the past.

4. BACK PAIN

Back pain is a common situation for many of my clients. That's not unusual—some studies report that as many as four out of five people experience symptoms. It can stem from an injury that did not heal properly, poor posture while sitting or standing, heavy lifting, or repetitive activities while the body is out of balance. Pain typically results from spinal misalignment, muscle spasms and tension, nerve impingement, and inflammation of the soft tissues. Try my Backstage Alternatives to reduce pain/inflammation, soothe your muscles, and speed healing:

NOURISH AND HYDRATE. Bolster your diet with foods high in omega-3s like wild fish, walnuts, flaxseed, and chia seeds, as well as magnesium such as leafy greens and dark chocolate. Avoid sugar and wheat products, which cause inflammation. Drink 8–10 glasses of water and herbal tea per day.

SUPPLEMENT. Reduce pain/inflammation, soothe muscles, and repair damage with bromelain (200 mg daily), flaxseed oil (1 tablespoon daily), magnesium malate (300–500 mg daily), and vitamin C (1,000 mg daily). Herbs that work for inflammation and pain include boswellia, ginger, rosemary, turmeric, and white willow bark.

TREAT. Daily Epsom salts baths are the most affordable and immediate ways to soothe sore muscles and relieve pain. I also recommend weekly acupuncture, chiropractic manipulation, and deep-tissue massage treatments. Iyengar and hatha yoga are also great for alignment. If there's no studio nearby, look for free or low-cost classes online. Add physical therapy as needed.

5. CARPAL TUNNEL SYNDROME (AKA KEYBOARD WRIST)

You don't have to be a world-class guitar player or pianist to have carpal tunnel syndrome. It's one of the most common workplace injuries, thanks to excessive computer use. Put simply, the condition results from a narrowing of the carpal tunnel in your wrist, which causes the median nerve to be compressed. Symptoms include wrist pain with numbness and tingling of the fingers.

Try my Backstage Alternatives to reduce pain/inflammation, soothe your muscles, and repair damage:

NOURISH AND HYDRATE. Add bone-based broths and soups, which are high in ligament-healing minerals. Avoid foods that contain yellow dyes because they deplete vitamin B_6 and eliminate gluten and sugar, which cause inflammation and can exacerbate pain. Don't forget to drink 8–10 glasses of water and herbal tea per day.

SUPPLEMENT. Reduce pain and inflammation, soothe muscles, and repair damage with daily proteolytic enzymes with bromelain, magnesium malate (300–500 mg daily), omega-3 or flaxseed oil (1 tablespoon daily), and vitamin B_6 (50 mg daily).

"Going raw vegan seven years ago completely reversed carpal tunnel syndrome. I had it so bad I could not lift a plate. It's one hundred percent gone now. No chiropractic visits. No surgeries. The vegan lifestyle also got rid of insomnia, arthritis, and a variety of anxiety issues I had."
—SHARE ROSS, BASSIST, VIXEN

TREAT. Weekly acupuncture and chiropractic manipulation treatments for your wrist, elbow, and neck can alleviate pain and speed healing. If you're at an office, ask for an ergonomics evaluation of your workstation and check your desk at home to ensure correct posture and position. Wear wrist splints while working and sleeping for stabilization. Add physical therapy as needed.

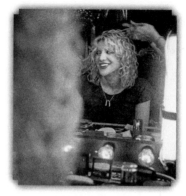

COURTNEY LOVE
(DANNY CLINCH)

6. CELLULITE

Cellulite technically isn't a "condition." It's a cosmetic "defect" of the fat in the subcutaneous layer of the skin that leads to a dimpling or mattress appearance in the thighs and buttocks. Toxins, poor circulation, dehydration, and water retention can worsen the situation. It's more prevalent in women and often causes quite a bit of psychological stress, especially for those under the paparazzi lens.

> "It is really quite important in rock & roll to, like, just be skinny. You can be a crackhead, but you can't be fat. You can lose all your hair, but you can't be fat. You can, and I have done this, go to the Bowery Ballroom the day after getting arrested, have laryngitis, no voice at all, and get a pornographic review in the *New York Times*, even though not one noise came out of your larynx, but you can't be fat!"
> —COURTNEY LOVE, SINGER, SONGWRITER, MUSICIAN

Try my Backstage Alternatives to increase your circulation, flush toxins, and minimize the signs of cellulite:

DETOX. The detox facilitates weight loss and body composition changes.

NOURISH AND HYDRATE. Eat foods that lower inflammation and reduce toxins, such as asparagus, cucumber, grapefruit, dark leafy greens, seaweed, and kelp. Avoid saturated fats, sugar, refined carbohydrates, sodas, artificial sweeteners, and alcohol, toxins that can exacerbate the condition. Staying hydrated flushes toxins and reduces the appearance of bumps and dimples. Drink 8–10 glasses of water with freshly squeezed lemon or lime plus 1–2 cups of green tea, a natural detoxifier.

SUPPLEMENTS. Stimulate collagen production, increase circulation, and lower inflammation with gotu kola (30 mg daily), horse chestnut (500 mg daily), kelp or seaweed (daily, per bottle instructions), and vitamin C (1,000 mg daily).

TREAT. Massage argan oil into affected areas. My favorite product is Slenderize by Moroccan Elixir, which contains essential oils of grapefruit, sage, lemon, and basil.

You can also minimize signs of cellulite with weekly body wraps, sauna, and steam (20 minutes, 3 times weekly), exercise (30 minutes of aerobic exercise daily), skin brushing (5–10 minutes daily in the shower), and weekly massage with essential oils of grapefruit, rosemary, juniper, and cedar.

7. COLDS AND FLUS

Both colds and flus are caused by viral infections of the upper respiratory tract, which may lead to sneezing, fevers, body aches, malaise, fatigue, and sore throat. Anyone traveling a lot, experiencing stress, sleeping too little, or otherwise living on the extreme end of the health spectrum is at risk. The best prevention is to keep your immune system strong. Try my Backstage Alternatives to strengthen your immune system:

DETOX. The detox is a great way to kick off cold and flu season. Keep drinking the shake once a day to enhance immunity.

NOURISH AND HYDRATE. Eat extra fruits and veggies that are yellow, orange, and red in color (they're filled with antioxidants) as well as food with antibiotic properties, such as garlic and onions. Avoid sugar, dairy, wheat, and alcohol, which are inflammatory and weaken your immune system. Finally, stay hydrated by drinking a minimum of 8–10 glasses of water and herbal tea, especially if you're already sick.

SUPPLEMENT. Boost immunity with probiotics containing *Lactobacillus acidophilus* (daily, per bottle instructions) and vitamins A (25,000 IU daily) and C (1,000 mg daily). Supplement with herbal cold and flu fighters like astragalus, echinacea, elderberry, goldenseal, and ligusticum. Try essential oil of eucalyptus and peppermint under the nose or in massage oil to soothe coughing and clear sinuses.

TREAT. Apply a nightly chest rub of eucalyptus oil or balm to ease coughing. Bolster your defense with acupuncture 1–2 times weekly. Finally, limit or avoid exercise while your body heals and be sure to sleep 8–10 hours a night.

8. CONSTIPATION

You probably don't need a detailed definition of constipation. It's a dilemma for many people and usually gets worse when you're traveling because your normal diet, sleep patterns, and daily rhythms are off. Naturopathic doctors consider it normal to have three bowel movements per day. Yes, that would make most of our population constipated. Beyond discomfort, irregularity increases toxicity, which leads to fatigue, digestion problems, and a weakened immune system. Try my Backstage Alternatives to get regular:

DETOX. The detox improves colon health and regularity.

NOURISH AND HYDRATE. Fill your diet with foods that aid digestion and promote regularity like ground flax seeds or chia seeds (1 tablespoon daily) as well as fiber-rich foods including fruits, vegetables, dark leafy greens, beans, and whole grains. Reduce dairy, gluten/wheat, sugar, and red meats, which cause irregularity, and be sure to drink 8–10 glasses of water daily to facilitate digestion.

SUPPLEMENT. Many of Mother Nature's remedies act as natural laxatives and aid digestion. I recommend: daily fiber powder supplements, high-lignin flaxseed oil (1 tablespoon daily), magnesium oxide (500 mg daily in the evening), daily probiotics with *Lactobacillus acidophilus*, and vitamin C (1,000 mg daily). Herbal laxatives can also be highly effective. Try cascara sagrada, chicory, dandelion, psyllium, red clover, turkey rhubarb, and yellow dock.

TREAT There are some simple things you can do at home to improve regularity.

For instance, abdominal massage in a clockwise direction—up the right side, across the middle, down the left—or yoga poses like spinal twists. Weekly acupuncture and daily exercise can also keep things moving.

NO SATISFACTION
••••••••••••••••••••

I joined a band in France while they were on their first European tour. There was a lot of tension, as the female lead singer was not getting on too well with her band-mates. After spending some time with her, I found that she was on her fourth day of touring in France while being constipated. She was quite miserable and told me the only food provided backstage was bread, cheese, and wine. No vegetables means no fiber. The buses were small and had miserable little toilets and the entire band was in one bus. The hotel rooms were barely large enough for one to walk in and the bathrooms were more suited for dollhouses. Not to mention the schedule was quite grueling. All of this added up to her unbearable situation.

I began giving her all the herbal laxatives and magnesium that I had with me. Two more days went by and no luck. Next, we hit up pharmacies for medical laxatives and enemas. Two more days, and nothing. By this time, she looked quite toxic. She had a very small frame and her belly made her look like she would soon be giving birth to a baby bread-and-cheese ball.

I was worried that things were getting dangerous, so I took her to a hospital. The doctor who examined her told us that nine days without going to the bathroom was not so bad, and for many people, it was normal. He gave her a laxative and sent us on our way, annoyed. As we took the taxi back to the hotel we speculated that if nine days without pooping is normal in France, maybe this is why the French have a reputation for being so crabby.

That night she tried the medical laxative, but the only thing it gave her was cramps and dry heaves. She rolled on the bathroom floor in agonizing pain. I spent the night sitting outside the bathroom door expecting her remains to be splattered all over the bathroom floor by morning. She was exhausted and crying.

I decided it was time to break out my darkest-secret remedy, the one that must always be saved for last. I shared my story of constipation in India: After nine days of no luck and every Ayurvedic treatment known to man, I discovered that two puffs of a cigarette brought me to enlightenment. One of the band members hand-rolled her a cigarette with American Spirit tobacco. It worked! She gave birth minutes after her first two puffs.

The entire band rejoiced with her. Unfortunately, she became dependent on the two puffs of a cigarette every night after the show for the rest of the tour. After the tour, I gave her a detox protocol and some acupuncture to stop the smoking. She easily quit smoking, but vowed never to tour Europe again!

9. DEHYDRATION

Dehydration is one of the most common nutritional deficiencies in the American diet. Most of us are not drinking enough water—you need to drink about half your body weight in ounces daily and not all liquids are created equal. One of my rock stars once asked if he could count beer ounces in his daily water allotment. Um, no. But you can count the electrolyte-rich fluids listed below. Symptoms of dehydration include: fatigue, constipation, dehydration, digestive problems, and many other issues. One way to know if you are dehydrated is by the color of your urine. It should be clear or a very light yellow. Try my Backstage Alternatives to hydrate and increase electrolytes:

HYDRATE. Drink 8–10 glasses of water or herbal tea daily along with miso soup or coconut water (add to your detox shake if you're detoxing). At the same time, limit caffeine intake to 2 cups daily. For each cup of caffeine you drink, increase your water intake by 2 cups to replace lost fluids.

NOURISH AND HYDRATE. Add electrolyte-rich vegetable bouillon or soups to your diet while increasing potassium-rich foods like bananas, apricots, avocados, and leafy greens.

SUPPLEMENT. Look for natural hydrators including: dehydrated coconut water (1 teaspoon daily); Emergen-C (1–2 packets daily in water); and potassium, calcium, and magnesium formulas (daily, per bottle instructions).

TREAT Enhance your water with electrolytes when traveling, detoxing, and exercising or during warmer weather or stressful times. And remember the desert survival rule at Burning Man: you're not hydrated until you piss clear.

10. DEPRESSION

"It ain't nothin' but the blues" can be a powerful mind-set to hold when you're feeling gloomy, down, or apathetic. Any number of factors can impact your mood, including poor diet, chemical imbalances, physical conditions, social and emotional situations, and spiritual deprivation. The blues, however, can turn into something far more serious when prolonged and untreated. If this happens, see your doctor, but in the meantime, there are some natural remedies that can improve your outlook on life.

> **"My mood can get low out on the road. I deal with that in two ways: I take medication that lifts depression, and I don't tour alone. I used to go on the road by myself and it was lonely and disorienting. So now, even if it's just me on the bill—and it usually is—I take my tour manager, Carolyn."**
> **—SHAWN COLVIN**, SINGER, SONGWRITER

Try my Backstage Alternatives to improve your mood and enhance brain function:

DETOX. Detoxing leads to a better mood through greater vitality.

NOURISH AND HYDRATE. Eat brain-boosting foods such as wild cold-water fish, eggs, coconut oil, olive oil, organic meats, dark chocolate, and dark leafy greens. Avoid sugar, alcohol, refined carbohydrates, sodas, and processed foods, which cause hormone and blood sugar imbalances that impact your mood and brain function. Dehydration can heighten anxiety by causing mood swings, fatigue, tension, and difficulty concentrating. Drink 8–10 glasses of water daily to stay hydrated and limit caffeine to 1–2 cups daily. Too much caffeine increases cortisol, which can cause depression and anxiety.

SUPPLEMENT. Increase neurotransmitters and improve brain function with 5-HTP (50–100 mg at dinner), daily B-complex vitamins, and L-tyrosine (50–100 mg in the a.m.). Add herbs with extra mood-boosting power including ashwagandha, maca, rhodiola, Saint-John's-wort (300 mg, 3 times per day), and Siberian ginseng.

TREAT. For more immediate relief use ylang-ylang essential oil, a natural antidepressant, in a diffuser in your home or office. Every day, exercise 20–30 minutes to boost serotonin levels, meditate 10–20 minutes, play or do something you love, and surround yourself with friends and family. Shoot for 8 hours of sleep each night and before bed, try Oprah's favorite trick: list five things you are grateful for to shift your focus to the positive things in your life. Reconnecting to your spiritual path can also move you out of negative feelings of self-worth, worry, or fears. Finally, I recommend weekly acupuncture, Reiki, and psychotherapy (or as needed) treatments to round out your daily treatments.

"I find that meditation coupled with a fair amount of physical exercise does wonders for many conditions, including depression and the loneliness of the road."
—JEFF PILSON, BASSIST, FOREIGNER

RAVE REVIEW

The scene is Glastonbury Music Festival, England. This massive music festival takes place on the summer solstice each year at the site of the ancient Stonehenge. Imagine numerous stages and campgrounds sprawled across nine hundred acres of private farmland. My first year working there was the year after the promoters built a large wall around the festival to deter the thousands of fans who would sneak in without a ticket. The Brits were very unhappy about the wall. As I drove in, I could see bulldozers and tractors full of fans trying to "Tear Down the Wall." Paying at Glastonbury was not an option!

I had a day to unwind before I started working so I spent an evening camping with friends in the massive tent village. The party scene was an experiment in British pharmacopeia. There were pills and more pills with every imagined combination of letters in the alphabet: MDA, GHB, DMA, Super K, and the list goes on. Fans were drinking down the pills with alcohol and Red Bull drinks. As the night went on, the debauchery got crazier and crazier.

Needless to say, I was relieved to start working. They assigned me to the DJ tent to work with the electronic music artists. I was able to help with things such as wrist and elbow tendinitis, a condition that comes from the repetitive movements involved in spinning records and such. Over the course of the week, several DJs confided that they suffered from insomnia, anxiety, and depression. Many were on prescribed medications and were mixing them with the party pills. I avoided using any herbs and supplements since I was fairly inexperienced with this scene and did not want to add to the chemical confusion in their bodies.

I befriended an American DJ who was interested in the natural medicine approach to his depression and insomnia. I told him to find me some time off tour and I would work with him. Two years later, he came to see me. Although he had stopped all the party pills, he was on several meds for depression, anxiety, and insomnia. He had stopped spinning because he had lost all interest in his music and had even contemplated suicide. The scene had really taken its toll on him physically, emotionally, and creatively.

He wanted to get off his meds and treat his conditions through natural therapies. I spent a year working with him and his psychiatrist. We started with general diet changes and detox. After he was cleaned out, he began rebuilding therapies to support his adrenal glands and neurotransmitters, along with intensive psychotherapy and regular acupuncture treatments. Within six months he felt really great, and we worked with his psychiatrist on a step-down protocol for the medications. Six months later, he was off the meds. After just one year of deep work physically, emotionally, and spiritually, he began creating and performing again. To this day, he's free of all meds and does no recreational drugs. And he feels that his music is even more creative now that he is clean!

11. FATIGUE

Fatigue is an American epidemic and may simply be the result of expending more energy than you take in. It can also be a red flag for more serious conditions. See your doctor to investigate the underlying cause and rule out poor diet, anemia, thyroid dysfunction, adrenal imbalance, gastrointestinal issues, toxicity, chronic stress, insomnia, and other systemic issues. Try my Backstage Alternatives to improve your mood and boost your energy:

DETOX. The detox leads to greater energy and vitality.

NOURISH AND HYDRATE. Add mood-boosting foods to your diet, including complex carbohydrates, such as whole grains, legumes, vegetables, nuts and seeds, organic meats, wild fish, and fruits. Eat several small meals or snacks daily with protein to keep energy up and avoid quick-fix pick-me-ups like caffeine, alcohol, sugar, white flour, artificial sweeteners, and soda. They'll simply spike your blood sugar and cause you to crash later. Drink 8–10 glasses of water daily to stay hydrated and enhance brain function.

SUPPLEMENT. Improve your mood and energy with a daily B-complex, CoQ10 (100 mg daily), L-carnitine (500 mg daily), L-tyrosine (100 mg in the a.m.), magnesium malate (500 mg daily with food), and omega-3 or flaxseed oils (1 tablespoon daily). Herbs that beat fatigue? Try Korean ginseng, licorice root, nettles, oatstraw, rhodiola rosa, and Siberian ginseng.

TREAT. Shoot for weekly sessions of acupuncture, massage, Reiki, and yoga along with 15–20 minutes of exercise a day. Keep essential oils of rosemary and basil, natural energizers, in a diffuser in your home and workspace. Finally, sleep 8–10 hours nightly so your body can rest and heal.

12. HEADACHES

Most of us associate headaches with stress, but they also can be caused by many other factors, including dehydration, low blood sugar, muscle spasms, jaw pain, neck misalignment, hormone imbalances, and poor diet. This is fairly common for people under immense pressure combined with strains of a busy lifestyle, irregular sleep, and more. By arming yourself with a few basic tools, you can reduce your risk of getting them and quicken your recovery. Try my Backstage Alternatives for pain relief:

DETOX. The detox balances hormones, reduces inflammation, and eases pain.

NOURISH AND HYDRATE. Reduce inflammation, pain, and muscle tension by avoiding sugar, alcohol, white flour, food dyes and additives, artificial sweeteners, and MSG. Enjoy dark chocolate if your headache is not a migraine. Drink 8–10 glasses of water daily, along with caffeinated coffee or green tea and ginger tea, a natural anti-inflammatory.

SUPPLEMENT. Reduce inflammation, pain, and muscle tension naturally with daily B-complex vitamins, bromelain and proteolytic enzyme formulas (daily, per bottle instructions), magnesium malate (500 mg daily), and omega-3 or flaxseed oils (1 tablespoon daily). Herbs that further support relief include boswellia, feverfew, ginger, turmeric, and white willow bark.

TREAT. Weekly acupuncture, chiropractic manipulation for neck alignment, cranial sacral therapy, massage, and yoga can reduce the frequency and severity of headaches. Be sure to sleep 8–10 hours a night. Stress on the mind and body only makes headaches worse. When you're experiencing pain, apply essential oils of lavender, peppermint, and rosemary to temples and forehead.

13. HEARTBREAK AND GRIEF

While they're the inspiration for many a great rock song, in reality heartbreak and grief can lead to emotional and physical symptoms, such as depression, anxiety, insomnia, and more. Try these Backstage Alternatives to ease grief, fight depression, and boost mood:

NOURISH AND HYDRATE. Enjoy dark chocolate as well as dark-skinned fruit and berries, wild fish, raw nuts, and seeds. Avoid sugar, soda, white flour, alcohol, and artificial sweeteners, which are toxins that can exacerbate symptoms. Drink naturally calming herbal teas of passionflower, chamomile, and hawthorn.

SUPPLEMENT. Ease grief, fight depression, and boost mood with daily B-complex, magnesium/calcium supplements (500 mg/500 mg nightly before bed), omega-3 or flaxseed oils (1 tablespoon daily), and Rescue Remedy (5 drops, 3 times daily). Herbal remedies include hawthorn berries, passionflower, and rosehips, while homeopathic remedies include Ignatia 12X and Natrum muriaticum 12X.

TREAT. Weekly acupuncture, massage, and psychotherapy to ease symptoms. Be sure to get 8–10 hours of sleep nightly and connect with friends and family daily. Chest-opening yoga poses can also boost your mood and open your heart.

14. HEARTBURN

Nothing screams heartburn, reflux, and stomachaches like road trips, diners, coffee fixes, smoke breaks, and happy hours, all-too-common occurrences in a rock star lifestyle. Digestive problems result from unhealthy diets, toxic environments, alcohol, caffeine, nicotine, poor digestive function—all the things that live in the 10 percent of the 90/10 Rule—and in some cases, a bacterial infection called *Helicobacter pylori*.

HARM REDUCTION TECHNIQUE: DON'T REFILL YOUR GLASS AT DINNER

Limit water to one glass at meals. Too much fluid can dilute the digestive enzymes, preventing you from digesting your food well.

Try my Backstage Alternatives to heal and protect the GALT:

DETOX. The detox strengthens the stomach and digestive system.

NOURISH AND HYDRATE. Eat easily digestible foods such as white rice, yogurt, oatmeal, and cooked foods. Enjoy smaller meals more frequently instead of large meals so you don't overeat and don't forget to chew your food well. Drink 8–10 glasses of water a day, but avoid drinking at the same time as you eat because it dilutes the enzymes.

Finally, avoid caffeine, alcohol, sugar, spicy foods, tomatoes, citrus, and white flour, which can trigger heartburn.

SUPPLEMENT. Heal and protect the GALT with glutamine (1,500 mg daily), daily probiotics, and digestive enzymes (1 with each meal). Herbs are also helpful in treating heartburn. I recommend aloe, deglycerinated licorice, marshmallow, okra, and slippery elm.

TREAT. Alternative therapies work well for heartburn. I recommend: weekly acupuncture, chiropractic manipulation of the thoracic spine, weekly Rolfing sessions to release diaphragm tension, adjusting your posture for proper and lifted alignment, 8–10 hours of sleep nightly on a slant with head and upper body elevated, and chest-opening yoga poses, like back bends, that expand the front of the body and release the stomach.

15. HERPES

This sexually transmitted disease (STD) is a recurrent viral infection of the skin or mucous membranes that results from kissing, sexual intercourse, or skin-to-skin contact. Many people are carriers of the virus, but it lies dormant and does not cause symptoms. Outbreaks may follow emotional stress, sun exposure, infection, injury or trauma, and poor diet. Not all people exposed to herpes will contract it because each person's immune system is different. This means preventing the condition or its recurrence is possible using the remedies listed here. I also recommend them if you're having an active outbreak.

Try my Backstage Alternatives to strengthen your immune system:

DETOX. The detox boosts your immunity so outbreaks become less frequent and last fewer days. Follow with the shake for maintenance.

NOURISH AND HYDRATE. Reduce the severity and frequency of outbreaks by eating foods high in lysine, like cheese, eggs, chicken, fish, yogurt, avocado, figs, potatoes, lamb, and beets. Also, increase foods high in antioxidants, like fruits, vegetables, sprouts, and green tea. At the same time, avoid foods high in arginine (chocolate, nuts, seeds, and oatmeal), which can trigger outbreaks, as well as sugar, alcohol, caffeine, refined white flour, milk, and artificial sweeteners, which lessen your immunity. During outbreaks, eliminate acidic foods, like citrus fruits, because they can increase the severity. Finally, keep your body functioning at its peak by keeping it hydrated—drink 8–10 glasses of water a day especially during an outbreak.

SUPPLEMENT. Reduce the severity and frequency of outbreaks with daily antioxidants containing bioflavonoids, B_{12}/folic acid (1,000 mcg/800 mcg daily), L-lysine (1,000 mg, 3 times daily), omega-3 or flaxseed oils (1 tablespoon daily), vitamin C (2,000 mg daily), and zinc (25 mg daily). Herbal remedies can lessen the severity of outbreak. I recommend andrographis, echinacea, lemon balm, licorice root, and olive leaf. Topical remedies can also provide relief during an outbreak. Try aloe vera, calendula, chamomile, lemon balm, and licorice.

TREAT. Boost immunity and detoxification with weekly acupuncture treatments, yoga, and Epsom salt baths while reducing stress through daily meditation and exercise. During outbreaks or when fatigued, avoid over-exercise and be sure to get 8–10 hours of sleep per night. Soothe outbreak symptoms with ice, applied directly to the affected area. For additional symptom relief, add essential oils of basil, lavender, lemon balm, and rosemary to massage oil before applying.

SEXUAL HEALING

In the mid-eighties I was asked to massage a rock star from a heavy metal band. I was escorted backstage through an area where I saw a long line of girls waiting outside the artist's dressing room. I was told to wait for a while. There was a guy walking around with a walkie-talkie who was getting messages from the artist onstage. I found out that this guy's job was to go out into the audience and bring back the girls whom the artist wanted to have sex with. The artist would notify him about where she was and what she was wearing. It was very disturbing, even more so after seeing the girls' boyfriends waiting for them outside the backstage door after they slept with the artist. I spent an hour staring with disgust at the entire scene, trying not to judge, and taking as many water and bathroom excursions as I could to regroup.

Finally, I was asked to give the massage. I felt sick entering the dressing room. The artist wore spandex leopard pants, a vest with no shirt, and cowboy boots. His hair was long and stringy. Even in the eighties, this was a fashion "don't!" I told him he had to shower if he wanted me to work on him, so I left until he was ready for his treatment.

During the massage, the artist bragged about the girls. I told him that I thought he was sick, disrespectful, and foolish for not using protection during sex. He was annoyed at my lack of enthusiasm for his bravado. Obviously, he was not used to being around a woman who did not see his sex appeal.

Fifteen years later, I was working backstage at a music festival and the artist was there with his then fiancée. By this time he had a receding hairline and a beer belly and, thank God, no more spandex! He came to me to get an adjustment and massage, not remembering that I had worked on him many years before. When he found out that I was a naturopathic doctor, he asked me some questions regarding a problem he had—herpes.

I was hardly shocked, but glad to help. I offered him the natural remedies and dietary advice listed in this chapter to support his immune system and prevent outbreaks. He was grateful. I refrained, but all I could think was, "Told you so!"

16. HYPOGLYCEMIA

Hypoglycemia, or low blood sugar, may cause irregularities and swings in energy and mood that can negatively impact your daily life. Other symptoms include headache, irritability, depression, anxiety, blurred vision, weakness, and fatigue. Hypoglycemia is easily balanced with diet and lifestyle. It's seen in people who skip meals or eat too little, which is a common side effect of a rock star lifestyle. Unfortunately, continued irregularities in blood sugar may eventually lead to diabetes. Try my Backstage Alternatives to balance blood sugar:

DETOX. The detox helps balance blood sugar.

NOURISH AND HYDRATE. Eat high-fiber foods like beans, broccoli, leafy greens, apples, and dark-skinned berries and remember to pair them with high-quality protein to keep blood sugar levels from spiking. Adding more protein foods to your diet such as oatmeal, yogurt, eggs, nuts, and cheese can keep energy and mood levels from plummeting. Avoid sugar, alcohol, caffeine, soda, refined white flour, and artificial sweeteners, toxins that also cause blood sugar imbalances. Finally, drink 8–10 glasses of water daily.

SUPPLEMENT. Stabilize blood sugar levels with daily B-complex supplements, chromium (200–400 mg daily), omega-3 or flaxseed oil (1 tablespoon daily), daily fiber supplements, and whey protein (15 g daily). Herbs can also keep blood sugar balanced. Try dandelion, gymnema, licorice, nettles, and red raspberry leaf.

TREAT. Weekly acupuncture and massage help blood sugar levels remain balanced. Also shoot for 15–20 minutes of exercise daily and 8–10 hours of sleep nightly.

17. INSOMNIA

Insomnia, or poor sleep quality, is a major problem for anyone living the extremes of a work-hard, play-hard lifestyle. Poor sleep might seem harmless, but it does more than give you the yawns. Over time, it weakens your immunity and increases stress, weight gain, premature aging, depression, anxiety, and fatigue.

"In the past I've suffered from insomnia on the road and like most touring people, musicians, crew, etc., I have relied heavily on sleep aids, natural and prescription. I find that this can be so much more productively addressed with exercise, a good mental attitude, and not too much food before bed."
—BRANDI CARLILE, SINGER, SONGWRITER

Try my Backstage Alternatives to promote sleep:

NOURISH AND HYDRATE. Eat foods that promote sleep—oatmeal, yogurt, cheese, and turkey—and a protein snack, like eggs and nuts before bed to keep metabolism high. In the evening, avoid sugar, alcohol, chocolate, caffeine, and nicotine, stimulants that will keep you awake.

SUPPLEMENT. Boost serotonin, lower cortisol, and ease stress with magnesium glycinate (300–500 mg before bed), melatonin (3 mg before bed), omega-3 or flaxseed oils (1 tablespoon daily), phosphatidyl serine (50 mg before bed), and theanine (100 mg before bed). Herbal remedies that support sleep include ashwagandha, chamomile, hops, passionflower, skullcap, and valerian root.

TREAT. Promote sleep with weekly acupuncture and cranial sacral therapy treatments. Complement those remedies with chiropractic manipulation as needed, nightly Epsom salt baths, meditation before bed, and 20 minutes of sunshine daily without sunglasses.

Daily exercise also improves the quantity and quality of your sleep, as long as it's not within three hours of bedtime. Finally, unplug! Stop using all electronics 1–2 hours before sleep.

18. JET LAG

If you've flown across different time zones, you've likely experienced jet lag. When this happens, your body clock and rhythms get out of sync, causing issues with sleep, energy, mood, and hormone balance. Recovering quickly is essential for frequent travelers so their productivity and health will not be compromised from the constant movement. Try my Backstage Alternatives to combat jet lag symptoms:

NOURISH AND HYDRATE. Eat the proper meal for the new time zone even if it is a smaller one as well as a protein snack before bed, like oatmeal, yogurt, eggs, nuts, or cheese. Avoid sugar, alcohol, chocolate, caffeine, and artificial sweeteners, which can disrupt your sleep cycle and energy levels, and drink 8–10 glasses of water daily.

SUPPLEMENT. Boost neurotransmitters, energy, and electrolytes with Emergen-C (1–2 packets daily); Jet Zone homeopathic remedy before, during, and after the flight; melatonin (3 mg before sleep on the plane and for 3–7 days in the new time zone); and omega-3 or flaxseed oils (1 tablespoon daily). Herbs that promote sleeping? Hops, passionflower, skullcap, and valerian root. Also take herbs for stress: adaptogens, including ashwagandha, oatstraw, nettles, and Siberian ginseng.

TREAT. If possible, schedule an acupuncture appointment the days after flying, at your destination and at home. Sleep on the plane if it is the normal time for sleep as well as 8–10 hours in new time zone on arrival. Even if you don't feel like it, try to exercise 15–20 minutes daily while you're traveling and when you return. To help you relax, meditate 15 minutes before bed and turn off all electronics 1 hour before sleeping. Finally, get your UV rays. I recommend 20 minutes daily without sunglasses.

19. NECK PAIN/WHIPLASH (AKA HEADBANGER'S NECK)

Rock stars and fans know the feeling the day after a concert of headbanging. While whiplash injuries are common among fans and guitar players alike, neck damage and pain can also result from poor posture, too much computer use, injuries and accidents, and reading in bed. This can lead to headaches, jaw pain, vision issues, ringing in the ears, dizziness, and arm pain and numbness. Try these Backstage Alternatives to reduce inflammation and speed healing:

NOURISH AND HYDRATE. Eat magnesium-rich foods, such as dark chocolate, dark leafy greens, nuts, and legumes as well as those high in omega-3s, like flaxseed oil, wild fish, and chia seeds. Decrease inflammatory foods—sugar, alcohol, white flour, and milk—and be sure to drink 8–10 glasses of water daily.

SUPPLEMENT. Reduce pain and inflammation while speeding healing with bromelain (50 g daily), glucosamine sulfate (1,500 mg daily), magnesium malate (500 mg daily), and omega-3 and flaxseed oils (1 tablespoon daily). Add herbs like boswellia, myrrh, and rosemary for inflammation and kava-kava to relax muscles.

TREAT. Schedule weekly acupuncture and massage sessions as well as a chiropractic evaluation and manipulation of the neck.

Cranial sacral therapy can also provide relief. Use a cervical neck pillow at night and/or during travel. Stretch morning and night, and take Epsom salt baths before bed. Be sure to get an ergonomics evaluation of your workstation to ensure proper posture and position.

20. PREMENSTRUAL SYNDROME (PMS)

For most women, PMS is a four-letter word. The condition is a compilation of more than 150 symptoms that manifest for a week or two before your period and may be due to hormone imbalance or other conditions, such as poor diet, stress, structural misalignment of the uterus and ovaries, neurotransmitter imbalances, thyroid dysfunction, anemia, and more. Symptoms include: headaches, cramping, bloating, depression, anxiety, insomnia, breast tenderness, mood swings, increased appetite, weight gain, and food cravings. Try my Backstage Alternatives to balance hormones and alleviate symptoms:

DETOX. The detox helps to balance hormones.

NOURISH AND HYDRATE. Ease symptoms by increasing magnesium-rich foods—dark chocolate, sunflower seeds, leafy greens, and wild-caught salmon—as well as protein like oatmeal, yogurt, eggs, nuts, and cheese. Add raspberries, apples, oranges, and dark leafy greens to your diet for pain relief. Finally, drink 8–10 glasses of water daily to flush toxins and prevent bloating.

SUPPLEMENT. Boost your serotonin levels, energy, and mood with 5-HTP (50 mg in the evening to increase serotonin), daily B-complex, daily calcium D-glucarate, daily calcium/magnesium (500 mg/500 mg before bed), evening primrose oil (1,000 mg daily, starting two weeks before your period), flaxseed oil (1 tablespoon daily), a daily food-based women's multivitamin and mineral supplement, a daily probiotic supplement (in the morning with food), and vitamin D_3 (1,000 IU before bed). Herbs can also help reduce a variety of PMS symptoms. Try black cohosh, cramp bark, curcuma, dong quai, ginger, vitex, and wild yam.

TREAT. I recommend a variety of therapies that can be used in conjunction with each other to reduce a number of PMS symptoms: acupuncture (weekly before your cycle starts), chiropractic manipulation of your lower back and sacrum, nightly Epsom salt baths, exercise (20 minutes daily), massage oils of lavender, geranium, and clary sage on the belly, Mayan Abdominal Massage for uterus health (15 minutes daily), meditation (daily, 15 minutes minimum), sleep (8–10 hours nightly), sunlight (20 minutes daily without sunglasses), and yoga (1–2 times weekly).

21. ROTATOR CUFF INJURY (AKA DRUMMER'S SHOULDER)

There are four shoulder muscles that attach to the humerus or arm bone and have the action of rotating the shoulder and keeping the arm stable in the shoulder socket. These muscles attach via tendons to the bone. Rotator cuff injury is a slight tearing of the tendons from the bone and can cause shoulder pain and limits in shoulder movement. If it continues on long enough, it can lead to frozen shoulder syndrome, which is very difficult to heal. Try these Backstage Alternatives to reduce pain and inflammation and speed healing:

NOURISH AND HYDRATE. Eat fruits, veggies, leafy greens, whole grains, legumes, cheese, nuts, and yogurt. Avoid sugar, alcohol, wheat, milk, artificial sweeteners, and caffeine. Drink 8–10 glasses of water daily.

SUPPLEMENT. Reduce inflammation, soothe muscles, and repair damage with a daily B-complex, daily proteolytic enzyme formulas with bromelain, glucosamine sulfate (1,500 mg daily), magnesium malate (500 mg daily), a daily mineral formula with trace minerals, omega-3 or flaxseed oils (1 tablespoon daily), and vitamin C (1,000 mg daily). Add herbs for inflammation, including boswellia, ginger, myrrh, and turmeric. Try the homeopathic *Arnica montana* 12X for muscle soreness.

TREAT. Add weekly sessions of acupuncture, Rolfing, and massage (using essential oils of peppermint, lavender, marjoram, basil, and frankincense) to shoulder and neck as well as chiropractic manipulation (neck and thoracic spine) and physical therapy.

22. STRESS MANAGEMENT

Stress is a heightened state of activity and engagement. There are both good and bad types of stress. When negative stress continues for long periods of time there can be wear and tear on your nervous system and endocrine system that impacts the entire body and your health. Some of the symptoms associated with prolonged and unrelenting stress are anxiety, depression, fatigue, muscle tension, headaches, digestive problems, insomnia, and interpersonal issues with friends, family, and work.

Like I said in the beginning of this book, what is common is very different from what is normal. There are many natural and alternative remedies to reduce and alleviate the symptoms. Try my Backstage Alternatives to lower stress and improve brain function:

NOURISH AND HYDRATE.   Increase protein, fruits and veggies, and dark leafy greens with meals, while avoiding toxins like alcohol, sugar, caffeine, refined white flour, and artificial sweeteners. Be sure to drink 8–10 glasses of water or herbal tea daily.

SUPPLEMENT.   Reduce cortisol, increase serotonin, and calm anxiety with 5-HTP (50 mg daily), B-complex daily (in the a.m., per bottle dosage), magnesium glycinate (500 mg daily), omega-3 or flaxseed oils (1 tablespoon daily), theanine (100 mg daily), tyrosine (100 mg daily), and vitamin C (1,000 mg daily). Add herbal adaptogens for stress like ashwagandha, ginseng, licorice root, maca, nettles, oatstraw, rhodiola rosa, and Siberian ginseng.

TREAT.   Daily acupressure on the ear, forehead, or temple (it's even better when you can convince someone else to do it for you), along with weekly acupuncture, cranial sacral therapy, massage, Reiki, yoga, and coaching or therapy sessions. Exercise and meditate a minimum of 15 minutes each daily as well as spend time with friends and family. Nightly Epsom salt baths just before bed will help you calm before sleep.

23. TENNIS ELBOW (AKA DRUMMER'S ELBOW)

Tennis elbow is a tendinitis or sprain of the muscles of the forearm extension and not just for tennis stars and heavy metal drummers anymore. Any repetitive motions can cause this condition: drumming, strumming, computer work, sports, or injuries from carrying heavy things (toddlers included). Try my Backstage Alternatives to ease pain/inflammation and speed healing:

NOURISH AND HYDRATE. Increase cheese, yogurt, protein foods, fruits, veggies, and dark chocolate while avoiding sugar, alcohol, wheat, milk, soda, artificial sweeteners, coffee, and black tea. Don't forget to drink 8–10 glasses of herbal tea and water daily.

SUPPLEMENT. Ease pain/inflammation and speed healing with glucosamine sulfate (1,500 mg daily), magnesium malate (500 mg daily), a daily mineral formula with trace minerals, omega-3 or flaxseed oils (1 tablespoon daily), a proteolytic enzyme formula with bromelain (50 mg daily), and vitamin C (1,000 mg daily). Add herbs for inflammation, including boswellia, ginger, myrrh, turmeric, and valerian root. Try the homeopathic *Arnica montana* 15X for muscle soreness.

TREAT. Alternate hot and cold (10 minutes of each, always ending with cold), chiropractic manipulation (neck, thoracic, and arm joints), deep-tissue massage (extensor muscles of the arm), essential oils for massage (peppermint, basil, marjoram, frankincense, and lavender). Also, be sure to rest the area and use an elbow splint to stabilize the joint. Add physical therapy as needed.

24. THROAT CONDITIONS (AKA SINGER'S THROAT)

Sore throats, raspy voice, laryngitis, polyps, and more are common not just with rock stars, but also with public speakers, call center workers, mothers, teachers, and others who use their voice frequently. Try my Backstage Alternatives to ease symptoms and promote healing:

NOURISH AND HYDRATE. Increase your fruits and veggies and avoid alcohol, sugar, wheat, refined flour, artificial sweeteners, and dairy, which can increase inflammation and pain. Even if you're getting 8–10 glasses of water daily, increase your intake of water and herbal teas.

SUPPLEMENTS. Reduce pain and inflammation, soothe your muscles, and repair damage with omega-3 or flaxseed oils (1 tablespoon daily), a daily food-based multivitamin mineral complex, a daily probiotic, glutamine (1,500 mg daily), vitamin A (25,000 IU daily), and vitamin C (1,000 IU daily). I also recommend a variety of herbal remedies for the throat, including licorice root, slippery elm, aloe vera, marshmallow, and okra.

TREAT. Add any or all of the following treatments to ease throat issues: weekly acupuncture, breathing exercises, chiropractic manipulation of the neck, weekly cranial sacral therapy, neck and head massage, meditation (15 minutes minimum daily), sleep (8–10 hours nightly), stop smoking, voice therapy as needed, and chest-opening yoga postures. You can also uses essential oils like basil, lavender, myrrh, peppermint, and rosemary.

25. TINNITUS AND HEARING LOSS

Tinnitus is also known as ringing in the ears. It varies from person to person in terms of pitch, duration, and intensity. There

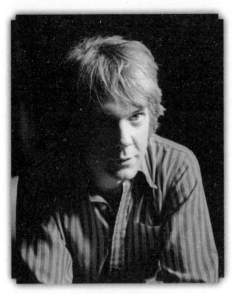

DAVE PIRNER
(DANNY CLINCH)

are many causes of tinnitus that should be evaluated by your doctor. Tinnitus can be caused by medications, head injury, loud music exposure, hearing loss, TMJ dysfunction, and certain diseases of the arteries and nerves related to the ears.

Hearing loss can be caused by a variety of reasons such as aging, illness, nerve damage, medications, injury, and of course loud noises.

Both hearing loss and tinnitus are common among rock stars, the band's crew, and of course the concertgoing fans. Besides loud concerts, many people are seriously damaging their hearing by listening to loud music in their headphones.

The best therapy for tinnitus and hearing loss is prevention.

"I went into depression because I thought that I was going deaf and I couldn't hear music anymore. So I came to New York to see the grand wizard of hearing. Loud music is an occupational hazard. The doctor was, like, turn it down, dumb shit! We put a piece of Lucite around the drum kit in order to bring the volume down onstage. I also did acupuncture and cranial sacral massage to help the stress and heal the inner ears. Now I protect my hearing all the time."

—DAVE PIRNER, SINGER, SONGWRITER, GUITARIST, **SOUL ASYLUM**

Try my Backstage Alternatives to ease symptoms and promote healing:

NOURISH AND HYDRATE. Get your omega-3 from fish oil and flaxseed oil; get magnesium from dark, leafy greens and chocolate; add some antioxidants with fruits and veggies; drink 8–10 glasses of water daily; and avoid caffeine, sugar, and alcohol.

SUPPLEMENTS. Decrease inflammation and restore function of cilia of the inner ear with daily supplements of omega-3 sources such as flax or fish oils (1 tablespoon), vitamin D (1,000 IU), B-complex (as prescribed on the bottle), B_{12}/folic acid sublingual (as recommended on the bottle), antioxidant formulas (as recommended), and zinc picolinate (90 mg). Helpful herbs for hearing loss and tinnitus are ginkgo biloba, rosemary, garlic, and plantain.

TREAT. Have chiropractic manipulation of the cervical spine, acupuncture, Eustachian tube drainage massage, and cranial sacral therapy once a week.

Prevent hearing loss by using earplugs at concerts, festivals, bars, and other loud places. Keep your mp3 player on a lower level, under 85 decibels.

SOUND RULES!

Kiss front man, Paul Stanley, has been a huge activist and advocate for educating young people about hearing loss and how it can be prevented. He says that nearly one in five teenagers now suffers from hearing loss, and that its primary cause is listening to loud music. His best advice for protecting your ears is to use earplugs at concerts and keep the mp3 below 85 decibels. Next time you go to a Kiss concert . . . get your earplugs in and "shout it out loud!"

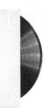

BONUS TRACKS

"I believe that if we listen to our bodies, we can sense the proper nutritional pathway to wellness. When we are beset with such conditions, I always seek a natural remedy through diet. The next phase, if necessary, might be a natural supplement or herb that specifically targets whatever issue I might have. When all else fails, I hit up the AMA and 'smart bomb' the crap out of my illness."

—KANE ROBERTS, GUITARIST, **ALICE COOPER**

"Music is therapy for people who have physical pain and, of course, mental pain. . . . I think that my love for music and how happy it makes me put my pain in another place. And taking narcotics is just blinding. You're blinding yourself from the pain."

—TRAPPER SHOEPP, SINGER, SONGWRITER, GUITARIST,
TRAPPER SHOEPP AND THE SHADES

"I use my Neti pot a lot on tour to prevent both allergies and infections."

—NINA ELISABET PERSSON, SINGER, SONGWRITER,
THE CARDIGANS

"Chiropractic, yoga, and massage are my fixes for my chronic back pain. Being pain-free allows for real enjoyment of playing and performing, rather than being in pain doing something I should be enjoying."

—DAVE ELLEFSON, BASSIST, **MEGADETH**

"My mother was a big proponent of natural and preventive therapies. She taught me to build my immune system at the first sign of trouble. For instance, when I feel the first tickle of a cold coming on, I take a traditional Chinese herb called yin qiao. I have averted many colds by using it the moment I start to feel unwell."

—DARRYL JONES, BASSIST, **ROLLING STONES**

"I try to eat primarily to my Ayurveda body type, which is mostly vata. Cooked foods, not too much sugar, nothing difficult to digest. I have chronic constipation. Yoga and diet make it better. Being on the road always makes it worse because of the irregularity of everything."

—JOAN WASSER, SINGER, SONGWRITER, KEYBOARDIST, VIOLINIST,
JOAN AS POLICEWOMAN

"I have struggled with jet lag. When you go to Europe, you often fly at night. So I try to stay up that first day, even if I haven't slept that well on the plane. If you go to the hotel and sleep, you are doomed. That first day is the key. You've really got to push yourself to go to bed at ten or eleven that night just to get over the daylight hump."

—GREG "WIZ" WIECOREK, DRUMMER,
NORAH JONES, AUTUMN DEFENSE, GOLDEN SMOG

"After my wife died of cancer, I didn't play music for almost seven months. My soul felt disconnected. I needed time to rebuild myself and reclaim my spirit. When I decided to go back on tour I chose to surround myself with choice people. It was the emotional support of the people around me that helped me to rebuild my life."

—CHARLEY DRAYTON, DRUMMER, BASSIST, PRODUCER, FIONA
APPLE, NEIL YOUNG, KEITH RICHARDS, DIVINYLS

"I've been to a voice doctor in Nashville and he was, like, here's the deal, dude, you got acid reflux. That's bad for your vocal cords, so take a Zantac. He said don't smoke, drink lots of water, and get enough sleep. These are three things that are totally impossible on tour. So now we have coconut water and we rehydrate ourselves more naturally. I mean, if you're a singer, you need liquid. You need to be moist."

—DAVE PIRNER, SINGER, SONGWRITER, GUITARIST,
SOUL ASYLUM

CHAPTER 12

ROCKERS AND RECOVERY

ADDICTION 101

Addictions are a sure way to sabotage a healthy rock star lifestyle. We live in a society plagued by addictions of all forms. In many ways the culture of our modern lives supports addictions and promotes them. This is truly an imbalance that has devastating effects on the balance of the body, mind, and spirit. Addictions are unique to each person and many of us can identify that we have an addiction of some kind. Addictions can be to caffeine, nicotine, sugar, food, love, work, the Internet, obsessive thinking, gambling, exercise, alcohol, drugs, and medications, to name a few. It is not necessary to judge one addiction as being worse than another. Once an addiction is recognized, it becomes quite consuming to the sufferer and is a central point of focus. The person becomes plagued by the physical symptoms and cravings as well as the emotional imbalances, guilt, and shame.

The decision to seek recovery from addiction is a very personal and individual one. Much of the time the awareness is brought on by the observations of friends, family, and coworkers. But admitting that you have the problem and being ready to work on it must come from within. The key to getting to this point is to not compare yourself to other people and their use. Recovery must be something that you want because what you have to lose from using is much greater than anything you have gained from it.

For many rock stars the choice of recovery was or is initiated by an intervention. I have seen this many times in bands where one member's partying has gotten so out of control, it disrupts the shows and the member's relationships with the band, their families, the promoters, and the production staff. Often the promoter threatens to cancel the tour if the abuse continues and the artist doesn't get clean. The decision becomes: treatment or tour? No tour means no money for the whole band. These days, artists are not making much money on records so the tour is the main income source. The pressure often becomes the wake-up call or rock bottom for artists who suddenly realize their behavior impacts not only them, but their families and the lives of everyone associated with the tour.

The 90-10 Rule is *not* an option for the majority of rock stars and non-rock stars who decide to recover from addiction because they've hit rock bottom. For most extreme people, the choice to heal involves "all or nothing."

It's also common for people to go from one addiction to another. They stop drinking and using drugs and then move into food, sugar, and nicotine addictions. They go from alcoholic to shopaholic to exercise-aholic to workaholic to sex-aholic. No matter your addiction, the twelve steps of recovery are the same and can be applied to help you heal emotionally and spiritually.

QUITTING TIME: WHEN ADDICTIONS AREN'T FUN ANYMORE

You can see and be "scene" without sacrificing your health. Some signs that your partying is no longer a good time:

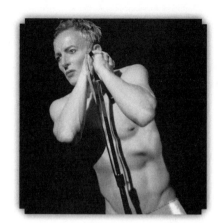

PHIL COLLEN OF DEF LEPPARD
(MICK ROCK)

- HANGOVERS THAT LAST A WHOLE DAY AND SOMETIMES MORE
- BLACKOUTS THAT YOU DON'T REMEMBER
- FIGHTS WITH FRIENDS AND FAMILY THAT ARE RELATED TO THE ADDICTION
- PROBLEMS GETTING/KEEPING WORK OR MAKING A LIVING
- FINANCIAL ISSUES RELATED TO THE ADDICTIVE BEHAVIOR
- LEGAL ISSUES: DUI, PUBLIC INTOXICATION, POSSESSION
- HEALTH COMPLICATIONS: DIABETES, WEIGHT GAIN, STOMACH ISSUES, LIVER PROBLEMS, COMPROMISED IMMUNE SYSTEM, OR PREMATURE AGING

"Now, I was a drinker back in the early days. It was totally acceptable, especially in hard rock music; the mantra was 'drinking is cool.' But I really didn't think it was cool, waking up and not remembering what I'd done, especially the driving part that really bothered me. I had to stop, cold turkey. Sobriety has given me a constant, inspired creative flow. Clear body, clear mind."

—PHIL COLLEN, GUITARIST, DEF LEPPARD

HITTING ROCK BOTTOM

One of the most important things about recovery, and this is something I learned when going through it myself, is not to compare your use to other people's. There will always be someone who looks wilder or crazier or more dysfunctional than you are. Knowing when to come clean is a very personal decision. Everyone's bottom is different. A lot of people think, "I only drink one day a week so that means I'm not an alcoholic." Or "I exercise excessively, but I still eat so I do not have an eating disorder." Or "I know this relationship is killing me, but I love him/her." And so on . . .

The real question to ask yourself: *What happens when I'm in addiction mode and how does it impact my life?*

If an addiction impacts your self-esteem, career, creativity, health, or relationships, it's a problem. It doesn't mean you're living in a gutter and sipping straight from the bottle all day. But if you have goals and an addiction is preventing them, it's time to come clean and find recovery.

For some people, this is rock bottom and enough to say, "I don't want this anymore in my life."

**IS IT TIME TO CHOOSE RECOVERY? ASK YOURSELF,
ARE ADDICTIONS NEGATIVELY AFFECTING MY:**

- Ability to make my dreams come true?
- Family?
- Health and well-being?
- Personal relationships?
- Self-esteem?

- Spiritual growth?
- Work life and career?
- Do I have a feeling a loss of control or powerlessness over the substance?
- Is there premeditated use?
- Do I need it to enjoy life or perform better?
- Do I crave it when I am not using it?
- Am I self-medicating?

TREATMENT OPTIONS: RECOVERY STARTS HERE

For help with addictions of all kinds there are twelve-step recovery groups. They provide a foundation and new paradigm for healing that revolves around a method of spiritual growth and community support. Twelve-step programs include:

- ALCOHOLICS ANONYMOUS
- NARCOTICS ANONYMOUS
- OVEREATERS ANONYMOUS
- FOOD ADDICTS ANONYMOUS
- SEX ADDICTS ANONYMOUS
- INPATIENT TREATMENT CENTERS
- OUTPATIENT TREATMENT CENTERS

The twelve steps were a spiritual awakening for me. The program includes a set of guiding principles for people going through addiction or any kind of crisis in life. Certain commitments are part of the pilgrimage: You admit that you don't have control over addiction; you recognize a higher power can give you strength; you admit past errors; you do an inventory of things you've done wrong when using; and you make amends (refer to aa.org for a listing of the entire twelve steps). You're sharing your issues with another person, and you've got a sponsor to connect with so you don't feel alone. These steps are rooted in most spiritual and religious traditions and innately part of human healing. And they're a metaphor for things other than addictions, including rebuilding relationships with people, with food, with exercise, with basically any issues you're battling.

In the music community they've begun sharing stories with fans because artists see the social responsibility that being an icon has for young people. If someone idolizes you but you're using drugs, that's not cool. Many bands that have gone through recovery will ask the venues where they are playing to not serve alcohol. This trend was very popular in the eighties and continues. It can be a disconnect for the artists to be in recovery when the audience is out of their minds.

COKE . . . IT'S THE REAL THING

Within a few minutes of entering the backstage of a huge stadium concert, the manager gave me the lowdown. The lead singer had been on a coke binge for several weeks. This had also taken its toll on the rest of the band and the entire tour. By this time, it had been three days since the singer had done any cocaine, but he was very edgy and having meltdowns. My job was to help him relax.

As we began his treatment, he told me that he was extremely agitated and tense all over. His facial muscles were so tight he was worried he wouldn't be able to sing well. I started to massage him and could feel the tension. As I was working, he reached over to his jeans and pulled out a container with some coke and a coke spoon. He gave each nostril a little snort and lay back down. I told him that this would counteract all the relaxation of the massage. He said that he was suffering from insomnia on the tour and needed just a wee bit of blow and coffee to give him energy for the show. Great, cocaine and coffee—the all-natural substitute for sleep! He made me promise not to tell the band, but it didn't matter, he had no idea what was coming for him.

The show was terrible. He was exhausted and his voice was hoarse. The band was furious and laid into him for ruining the concert. He stormed out of the after-party early and went back to the hotel. By the time the band and I arrived at the hotel, he had destroyed his room. Apparently, he had gotten in a fight with his wife on the phone and decided to take it out on the mirror and lamps. The band was kicked out of the hotel and forced to sleep in the tour buses. The manager and band were so upset that they started a fistfight with the singer and hotel manager. I was secretly kind of happy, because this was the first time in my entire rock & roll career that I had seen a hotel room torn up. I breathed a sigh of relief—this really was rock & roll!

I knew this was rock bottom. The tour ended. The band, the manager, and the artist's family held a drug intervention a couple of days later and the singer agreed to go into treatment. He checked himself into a twenty-eight-day treatment program to detox from drugs and alcohol.

The manager asked me to be part of the singer's post-treatment support. After he left the inpatient treatment, I used acupuncture for his cravings, detoxification for the years of abuse, and nutritional support to rebuild what was left of his adrenal glands. AA and NA were a great support for him. He took a year off to mend his relationships and get his health back. And soon he was back in the saddle, performing again.

THE RxSTAR RECOVERY PLAN

When I was younger and in a twelve-step program, it felt like staying clean was all about willpower. You have physical cravings that are hard to manage, so you go to a meeting, but the cravings don't go away. As I went through medical school and learned about the physiology behind addiction and cravings, I realized that when you work on the underlying physical and biochemical imbalances—at the same time you support yourself mentally and emotionally through the twelve-step program—recovery is easier. Addictions leave your body depleted and imbalanced, so when you use natural remedies for healing, the cravings go away, along with negative side effects from withdrawal. It's no longer a battle between you and your willpower.

In these recovery meetings, you'll see recovered addicts drinking massive amounts of coffee, shoveling down doughnuts, or chain-smoking, all of which give them speed-like effects. They've simply moved to other addictions: caffeine, sugar, nicotine. It's virtually impossible to have full healing if you're not treating the physical body as well.

Below you'll find my RxStar Recovery Plan, which includes pillars that should be considered when you're going through any type of addiction. It's designed to treat the underlying imbalances that occur during addiction so your physical symptoms lessen and you're more likely to succeed in handling the emotional and mental components of recovery.

f you have addiction issues, implement this program in conjunction with a doctor who can provide medical testing and a group that can offer emotional and mental guidance.

START WITH THE RxSTAR REMEDY DETOX

The detox is essential because it resets the system, cleans out residual toxins, gets the gut and liver back to ground zero, and creates a foundation for healing.

Change Your Diet

Eating nourishing food that serves as medicine supports healthy cell growth, balances hormones and blood sugar, and begins the rebuilding process.

Balance Blood Sugar

Many addictions are accompanied by blood sugar imbalance. When you drink, do drugs, or eat too much sugar, for example, it raises cortisol levels. This causes your body to secrete insulin to bring the stress hormone levels down. Insulin drops your blood sugar levels lower than they were before you indulged. That leads to cravings for something that will get you "high" again, whether it's caffeine, wheat, sugar, nicotine, or alcohol. Balancing blood sugar can help you get off the roller coaster of highs and lows that leads to constant cravings and mood swings.

Treat Candida Overgrowth

Candida is a normal flora yeast that lives in harmony with our probiotics or, good bacteria, on the lining of our digestive tract known as the GALT. When you drink too much alcohol or eat too much sugar, candida may grow out of control and turn into an "opportunistic infection." Candida overgrowth may cause relentless cravings for alcohol, sugar, and carbohydrates. To know if you have this, ask your doctor to be tested. Testing for candida is done by a stool culture or a parasitology panel. Symptoms include weight gain, puffiness in tissues, allergies, skin infections, gas and bloating, diarrhea, constipation, fatigue, sugar cravings, alcohol intolerance, frequent infections, and sinus congestion. And the list goes on.

Treating candida involves gut and immune support with some natural antifungal therapies. For many, it relieves the cravings for alcohol, carbohydrates, and sugar.

Balance Adrenal Glands and Hormones

The adrenal glands produce many types of hormones: stress hormones and neurotransmitters (epinephrine and norepinephrine); sex hormones (DHEA, estrogen, testosterone, progesterone); glucocorticoids (cortisol), which affect our blood sugar, inflammation, and immunity; and mineral corticoids (aldosterone), which regulate blood pressure and fluid balance.

Most addictions—drugs, alcohol, sugar, nicotine, and more—cause stress and depletion to your adrenal glands. Many doctors do functional adrenal testing through saliva and urine, which helps them recommend the appropriate nutritional and herbal supplementation to balance and restore adrenal health. Adrenal balancing is like recharging your batteries after they have been drained from years of abuse.

"I generally start by relaxing my breathing weeks prior. I am like a cruise ship; I start my engine slow and low for weeks. This is how I can control my adrenaline. When you're in Bad Brains, the music and expression are fast-paced and hyper-energetic, so controlling my adrenaline is key, especially at my age. I also try to eat a veg-based diet to cleanse my digestive system to prepare for the road and road food."

—DARRYL JENIFER, BASSIST AND FOUNDING MEMBER,

BAD BRAINS

Balance Neurotransmitters

Neurotransmitters are amino acid–based molecules that act as the communicating messenger between the nervous system, immune system, endocrine system, and gastrointestinal system. Some of the most famous neurotransmitters are serotonin, GABA, dopamine, adrenaline, norepinephrine, and phenylalanine. Medications for depression, anxiety, insomnia, and attention deficit disorders, for example, all affect these body-mind chemicals.

Neurotransmitter testing is an important tool in determining the baseline of your chemistry. I use Pharmasan Labs in Wisconsin to evaluate my patients who are suffering from post-addiction cravings, depression, anxiety, fatigue, and insomnia.

Targeted Amino Acid Therapy for Neurotransmitter Imbalance

Pharmaceutical drugs primarily work on neurotransmitters as reuptake inhibitors and receptor antagonists. This means that they prevent the absorption of the drugs on the cell receptors. This keeps the neurotransmitter in the blood longer, giving the effect of the chemical longer. Long-term use of these medicines may cause the true neurotransmitter levels to actually drop as the body stops producing them because it thinks that there is enough.

For example, if you take Lexapro for depression, the drug isn't raising your serotonin levels. It is keeping the serotonin in the blood, giving you the feel-good effects longer. But long-term use may lower your true levels and this in turn will create the need for more of the medicine to give you the same effect. That's why it's difficult to come off prescription drugs without feeling negative side effects.

The most effective natural therapy for neurotransmitter rebalancing is targeted amino acid therapy. It's my number-one treatment for clients in recovery. You discover through testing which specific chemicals are imbalanced and then give your body the building blocks—amino acids, vitamins, herbs, and minerals—so it can build up and manufacture more of these chemicals. Essentially your body rebalances itself with the support of this nutritional therapy. It is a very specific method of treatment and can best be employed with the help of a doctor who is trained to work with you. You can find a doctor who uses the testing and treatment by contacting www.neurorelief.com.

SELF-MEDICATING

Addicts often have an underlying chemical imbalance that they may be using food, substances, medicines, alcohol, or chemicals to self-medicate against. For example, someone low in adrenaline and norepinephrine naturally feels fatigued and unmotivated, so they will be drawn to stimulants like caffeine, speed, or cocaine. People low in serotonin and GABA will be attracted to alcohol, pot, or sedatives to calm them and help with anxiety. A person low in endorphins (our natural painkillers) produced by phenylalanine may be drawn to painkillers and narcotics. Those low in the pleasure molecule do-pamine seek out drugs like nicotine and cocaine. When neurotransmitters aren't balanced post-addiction, people may seek prescriptions for legal pharmaceuticals that give them the same effects the illicit drugs gave. Recovering coke addicts will feel blah and fatigued again, so they may seek caffeine or their doctor will write them an Rx for something like Ritalin. Often when people with neurotransmitter imbalances use drugs, they feel the way non-addicts feel when they are normal. The drugs are giving them a boost of something they are low in. However, long-term abuse of drugs and alcohol usually causes the chemical imbalance to become much worse. And the addict needs more to create the same effect as before.

Addictions may have devastating effects on our body, mind, and spirit. Awareness is the first step to healing addictions of all forms. It is often the wake-up call that initiates us on our path to health. There are endless resources for those suffering to find the help toward recovery of body, mind, and spirit. This book can barely touch the surface of what is available out there. But healing from addiction will always set your life in a new direction and help create a paradigm that supports the integration of a healthy lifestyle.

Join us on the adventure. . . .

"Don't drink if you have a bad relationship with booze. Everyone knows if they have a bad relationship with booze. I just got to the point where I was able to drink more than I should. I am not going to be the one sitting there having a beer ever, I am going to be the one having five beers always. And at some point, if that is your relationship to something after a long period of time, it is going to just turn sour. So it's time to move on."

—RUSSELL SIMINS, DRUMMER,

JON SPENCER BLUES EXPLOSION

"For years I was a drug addict rock star person that takes advantage of situations who is verbose and loud—we were put in that category. But if you sustain and live long enough, you discover that you're the farthest thing from that. What you are is an athlete."

—STEVEN TYLER, SINGER, SONGWRITER, MULTI-INSTRUMENTALIST,
AEROSMITH

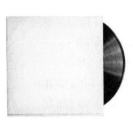

BONUS TRACKS

"I never abused myself with substances or alcohol. My first gig as a touring musician was with Ozzy Osbourne. Ozzy was my greatest teacher. When Ozzy would start drinking, it wasn't a few cocktails or a bottle. It was DAYS. I made a decision shortly into the first tour not to travel down that road. Otherwise, everything I'd worked for up to that point, you know, the rock & roll dream, would be thrown away. Wasted. I'm not a preacher. I believe that spirituality finds each person when he or she's ready. And when I said no to the alcohol and drugs, that was a spiritual decision."

—RUDY SARZO, BASSIST,
OZZY OSBOURNE, QUIET RIOT, WHITESNAKE

"I ended up in the ICU a day after my last record came out. I thought I was literally choking to death. I couldn't breathe or swallow! It was a crazy emergency and the doctors had to pump me up with steroids, Benadryl, and adrenaline-corporate drugs! Literally, my adrenal glands were not working! I felt very out of control in the hospital and with the doctors, none of them listened to anything I said. What helped me the most was to try to take some control— and I did this by shaving my head into a Mohawk when I was in Mexico. I felt like I had taken some control back. Taking control is what helped me!"

—CHAN MARSHALL, SINGER, SONGWRITER, CAT POWER

"I don't take drugs or alcohol anymore. I am a big comic book fan and I like to look at some of the comic book heroes. Some superheroes use their powers for only themselves. And other comic book heroes use their superpowers for the good of mankind and for the good of themselves and those around them. I have been both. I have been a self-destructive superhero who did not care about myself or anyone around me, and now I have superpowers to use for good."

—RICHARD MANITOBA, AKA "HANDSOME DICK," PUNK ROCK SINGER, THE DICTATORS

THE RxSTAR DETOX TEAR SHEET

U se this handy overview when you need a quick reference.

THE PROGRAM IS SIMPLE:

- The RxStar Detox Shake is a meal replacement for breakfast.
- Eat clean lunches, dinners, and snacks.
- Add more depth and power to your cleanse by incorporating body, soul, and lifestyle components.

RxSTAR DETOX SHAKE RECIPE

Functional food for liver (2 scoops, 15 g protein)

Intestinal repair powder (2 teaspoons)

Greens powder (1 scoop)

Probiotic powder (½ teaspoon)

Fiber powder (1 scoop)

Flaxseed oil (1 tablespoon)

Blend with 12–16 ounces of purified water.

Optional: Add ¼ cup of frozen organic berries or fruit as well as ¼ cup of yogurt, rice milk, almond milk, or soy milk.

Drink it in no less than 30 minutes—it is a meal.

SUPPLEMENTS

DIGESTIVE enzyme support for small intestines, pancreas—1 at lunch + 1 at dinner with food

LBS natural bowel stimulant—2 before bed with or without food

EMERGEN-C electrolyte replacement—1–2 packets per day with water

THE RxSTAR REMEDY SCAVENGER HUNT

Once you're finished with the RxStar Remedy Detox, don't slip back into old habits. Make life easy by rummaging through your kitchen for items that are bad for you and tossing them out. If junk food is your weakness, make a sweep for unhealthy foods every month or two. You're less likely to cheat if a bag of Cheetos isn't staring you in the face. Switch to natural body products—remember, what you put on your skin gets into the bloodstream.

Trash these babies (and recycle the containers, please):

Kitchen
Artificial sweeteners
Bottled water (plastic is bad for the environment)

Food dyes, colorings, preservatives, and additives
Genetically modified (GM) foods and irradiated foods
Hydrogenated and partially hydrogenated fats
Lunch meats with nitrates and nitrites
Monosodium glutamate (MSG)
Non-organic dairy
Non-organic eggs and chicken
Non-organic meats
Pasteurized cow's milk
Refined corn products (corn syrup, cornstarch)
Refined white flour foods (bread, pasta, pastries, cakes, cookies)
Refined white sugar foods (candy, cookies, cakes)
Soda and soft drinks (yes, diet versions, too)
Soy protein isolates (often hiding in the protein bars you're eating)
Vegetable oils that are not cold pressed or expeller pressed

Bath

Antiperspirants with aluminum
Body products with petroleum bases (PABA, paraben, methylparaben, petrolatum, mineral oil, sodium laurel sulfate)
Toothpastes with fluoride

Typically, at this point my clients say, "Holy &%$#@!!!! There is nothing left!!" Don't worry, an aggressive scavenger hunt gives you plenty of room to fill your kitchen and bath with the good stuff.

SPECIAL GUEST APPEARANCES

'm deeply grateful to all the incredible artists who shared their personal experiences and health regimens in *The Rockstar Remedy*.

A. Jay Popoff, singer, songwriter, drummer, LIT

Adrian Grenier, musician-actor-filmmaker-activist, Wreck Room, Honey Brothers

Angela McCluskey, singer, songwriter, Telepop, Wild Colonials

Amayo, singer-drummer, Antibalas

Ben Jaffe, upright bass and tuba, creative director Preservation Hall Jazz Band, awarded National Medal of Arts, 2006

Bess Rogers, singer, songwriter, Ingrid Michaelson Band

Brandi Carlile, singer, songwriter

Bill Sullivan, tour manager, Replacements, Soul Asylum, Bright Eyes, Cat Power, Jimmy Vaughn

Bridget Barkan, singer, songwriter, Scissor Sisters

Chan Marshall, singer, songwriter, guitarist, Cat Power

Charley Drayton, bassist, drummer, producer, Neil Young, Paul Simon, Keith Richards and the Expensive Winos,

Herbie Hancock, Johnny Cash, Rufus, Iggy Pop, Courtney Love, Simon and Garfunkel, and the Divinyls; producer, Fiona Apple

Conor Oberst, singer, songwriter, Bright Eyes, Los Desaparecidos

Courtney Love, singer, songwriter, musician

Craig Finn, singer, the Hold Steady

Danny Clinch, rock & roll photographer

Darryl Jenifer, bassist, Bad Brains

Dave Ellefson, bassist, Megadeth

Dave Navarro, guitarist, Jane's Addiction

Dave Pirner, singer, songwriter, guitarist, Soul Asylum

Del Stribling, aka "Binky Griptite," guitarist-emcee, Sharon Jones & The Dap-Kings

Ernie Cunningham, aka "Ernie C," lead guitarist, Body Count

Eve Jeffers, aka Eve, rapper-songwriter and producer

Fred Coury, drummer, Cinderella

Gabriel Roth, aka "Bosco Mann," bassist and songwriter, Sharon Jones & The Dap-Kings

Gary Louris, singer, songwriter, guitarist, the Jayhawks

Geoff Tate, singer-songwriter, Queensrÿche

Greg "Wiz" Wieczorek, drummer, Norah Jones, Autumn Defense, Golden Smog

Holly Miranda, singer, songwriter, musician

Ian Astbury, singer, songwriter, the Cult

Jeff Ament, bassist, songwriter, Pearl Jam

Jeff Pilson, bassist, Foreigner

Jenny Conlee, accordionist, the Decemberists, Black Prairie

Jennifer Finch, bassist, L7

Jessy Greene, violinist, Pink and Foo Fighters

Joe Satriani, instrumental rock guitarist

Joan Wasser, aka Joan as Policewoman, singer, songwriter, guitarist, violinist

John Waite, singer, songwriter

Jordan McLean, trumpeter, Fire of Space, Antibalas

Joseph Arthur, singer, songwriter, guitarist

Julia Haltigan, singer, songwriter, Julia Haltigan and the Hooligans

Kane Roberts, heavy metal guitarist, Alice Cooper

Kevin Cronin, singer, guitarist, REO Speedwagon

Kim Gordon, bassist, songwriter, producer, artist, Sonic Youth

Kirk Douglas, guitarist, the Roots

Kraig Jarret Johnson, singer, songwriter, guitarist, Jayhawks, Golden Smog, Joseph Arthur, Iffy, Run Westy Run

Liberty Devitto, drummer, the Slim Kings, Billy Joel

Lydia Lunch, singer, poet, author, actress, *The Need to Feed*

Máiréad Nesbitt, fiddler and violinist, Celtic Woman

Mark Batson, producer, multi-instrumentalist, songwriter, Dave Matthews Band, Dr. Dre, Eminem, 50 Cent, Alicia Keys, Nas, Marroon 5, Beyoncé, James Blunt; film composer, *Miami Vice, Beauty Shop,* and *American Hustle*

Mark Ronson, artist, DJ, producer, Amy Winehouse, Lily Allen, Bruno Mars, Sir Paul McCartney

Michael Stipe, singer, songwriter, R.E.M.; Rock and Roll Hall of Fame inductee

Mike D (Diamond), rapper, songwriter, drummer, producer, Beastie Boys, Rock and Roll Hall of Fame inductee

Mike McCready, guitarist, singer, songwriter, Pearl Jam

Mick Rock, rock & roll photographer

Mike Mills, bassist, singer, songwriter, R.E.M.; Rock and Roll Hall of Fame inductee

Mike Watt, bassist, the Minutemen, Firehose, Iggy Pop and the Stooges

Mike Wilbur, saxophone, Moon Hooch

Ori Kaplan, saxophonist, Balkan Beat Box

Orianthi, singer, songwriter, guitarist

Pat Sansone, keyboards, Wilco

Paul Cantelon, pianist, violinist, Wild Colonials; film
   composer, *Before Night Falls*, *Diving Bell and the Butterfly*

Pearl Aday, singer, Mötley Crüe, Meat Loaf

Peter Buck, guitarist, songwriter, R.E.M.; Rock and Roll
   Hall of Fame inductee

Phil Collen, lead guitarist, Def Leppard

Raine Maida, singer, songwriter, Our Lady Peace

Richard Fortus, guitarist, Guns N' Roses

Richard Manitoba, aka "Handsome Dick," punk rock singer,
   the Dictators

Rickie Lee Jones, singer, songwriter, pianist

Roddy Bottum, keyboardist, songwriter, Faith No More,
   Imperial Teen

Rudy Sarzo, bassist, Ozzy Osbourne, Quiet Riot, Whitesnake

Russell Simins, drummer, Jon Spencer Blues Explosion

Sameer Bhattacharya, guitarist, Flyleaf

Saul Simon MacWilliams, keyboardist, Ingrid Michaelson;
   producer, the Lovely Light

Scott Ian, guitarist, Anthrax

Serj Tankian, lead singer, System of a Down

Share Ross, bassist, Vixen

Sharon Jones, singer, Sharon Jones & The Dap-Kings

Shawn Colvin, singer, songwriter

Steve Lukather, guitarist, Toto

Steve Jordan, multi-instrumentalist, drummer, guitarist,
   composer, musical director, producer, Sting, Eric Clapton,
   Neil Young, Keith Richards (as producer and as an
   Expensive Wino), John Mayer; also veteran of Saturday

Night Live Band, the Letterman Band, the Blues Brothers
Band, the Grammys and the Oscars
Steve Riley, drummer, LA Guns
Steven Tyler, singer, Aerosmith; Rock and Roll Hall of Fame
inductee
Tim Booth, lead singer, James
Tommy Lee, founding drummer, Mötley Crüe
Trapper Shoepp, singer, songwriter, guitarist, Trapper Shoepp
and the Shades

CREDITS

INTERVIEWS CONDUCTED BY JULIE PANEBIANCO: Angela McCluskey, Ben Jaffe, Bill Sullivan, Chan Marshall, Charley Drayton, Conor Oberst, Courtney Love, Craig Finn, Danny Clinch, Darryl Jenifer, Dave Pirner, Gary Louris, Greg "Wiz" Wieczorek, Ian Astbury, Jenny Conlee, Jennifer Finch, Jessy Greene, Joseph Arthur, Kim Gordon, Kirk Douglas, Kraig Jarret Johnson, Lydia Lunch, Mark Batson, Mark Ronson, Mike D, Mike McCready, Mick Rock, Mike Mills, Mike Watt, Pat Sansone, Paul Cantelon, Peter Buck, Richard Fortus, Richard Manitoba aka "Handsome Dick," Rickie Lee Jones, Roddy Bottum, Russell Simins, Steve Jordan, and Trapper Shoepp.

INTERVIEWS CONDUCTED BY LONN M. FRIEND: Dave Ellefson, Dave Navarro, Ernie Cunningham, Fred Coury, Geoff Tate, Jeff Pilson, Joe Satriani, John Waite, Jordan McLean, Kane Roberts, Kevin Cronin, Orianthi, Pearl Aday, Phil Collen, Raine Maida, Rudy Sarzo, Scott Ian, Serj Tankian, Share Ross, Steve Lukather, Steve Riley, Steven Tyler, and Tommy Lee.

INTERVIEWS CONDUCTED BY STACY BAKER MASAND AND GABRIELLE FRANCIS: A. Jay Popoff, Adrian Grenier, Amayo, Brandi Carlile,

Bridget Barkan, Del Stribling aka "Binky Griptite," Eve Jeffers aka "Eve," Holly Miranda, Joan Wasser, Julia Haltigan, Máiréad Nesbitt, Mike Wilbur, Nina Elisabet Persson, Ori Kaplan, Sameer Bhattacharya, Saul Simon MacWilliams, Sharon Jones, Shawn Colvin, and Tim Booth.

RESOURCES AND INFORMATION

ALCOHOLICS ANONYMOUS (AA), aa.org

A resource for people who want to stay sober. Also see similar programs: Overeaters Anonymous (oa.org) and Narcotics Anonymous (na.org).

AL-ANON, al-anon.org

A resource for friends and families of alcoholics.

ALLIANCE FOR A HEALTHIER GENERATION, healthiergeneration.org

A group dedicated to fighting childhood obesity.

AMERICAN ASSOCIATION OF NATUROPATHIC PHYSICIANS (AANP)

APOTHE-CARRY NATURAL REMEDY KITS, apothe-carry.net

Wellness, prevention, and healing remedies, including essential oils, vitamins, topical treatments, herbal and homeopathic medicines for a variety of conditions and issues.

ARVIGO TECHNIQUES FOR MAYA ABDOMINAL THERAPY, www .arvigotherapy.com

Learn at-home techniques developed by Dr. Rosita Arvigo, based on ancient Mayan healing in Central America.

CROSSROADS CENTRE ANTIGUA, crossroadsantigua.org
Eric Clapton's nonprofit recovery facility for people in various stages of recovery. Set in the Caribbean to increase tranquility, privacy, and anonymity.

DO IT FOR THE LOVE FOUNDATION, doitforthelove.org
Michael Franti's wish-granting foundation, which helps people with advanced illness attend live concerts.

DR. GABRIELLE FRANCIS, theherbanalchemist.com
Sign up for a newsletter, download information, shop for the full line of RxStar Shakes, health products, and organic beauty.

EARTH EASY, eartheasy.com
Discover nontoxic, eco-friendly solutions for home and body.

EARTH 911-RECYCLING 101, earth911.org
A site that shares innovative ideas and advice on reducing waste.

EAT REAL, eatreal.org
Provides certification to restaurants that meet nutrition and sustainability benchmarks.

ECOLOGO, ecologo.com
Find certified green products and services for your home.

ENVIRONMENTAL WORKING GROUP, ewg.org
Calculate your exposure to toxins and learn how to reduce toxicity in your life.

EXERCISE APPS I LOVE:
- Gym Goal ABC
- Gym Guyz
- I Street Dance
- iTreadmill
- Lose it
- Run Keeper
- Pocket Salsa

FARM AID, farmaid.org
For three decades, this organization has supported family farming.

GAYE NELSON, gayenelson.com
A Los Angeles–based astrologist and tarot card reader.

GREEN DEPOT, greendepot.com
A resource for buying a variety of environmentally friendly products for your home.

GREEN MUSIC FESTIVALS
- Austin City Limits—Austin, Texas
- Beloved—Tidewater, Oregon
- Benicassim—Spain
- Bestival—British Isles
- Bonnaroo—Manchester, Tennessee
- Boom Festival—Idanha-a-Nova, Portugal
- Bumbershoot—Seattle, Washington
- Burning Man—Black Rock Desert, Nevada
- Byron Bay Bluesfest—Byron Bay, Australia
- Chicago Green Music Festival—Chicago, Illinois
- Coachella—Coachella Valley, California
- Croissant Neuf—changing locations

- Electric Forest Festival—Rothbury, Michigan
- Exit Fest—Vojvodina, Serbia
- Field Day—Sydney, Australia
- Forecastle—Louisville, Kentucky
- Friends of Nature Fest—Miami
- Fuji Rock Festival—Niigata Prefecture, Japan
- Glastonbury Festival—England
- Grassroots—Trumansburg, New York
- High Sierra—various spots in Northern California
- Hove Festival—Norway
- Lightning in a Bottle—Southern California
- Live Earth Concerts
- Lollapalooza—Chicago, Illinois
- Outside Lands—San Francisco, California
- Oya Festival—Norway
- Paleo Festival Nyon—Switzerland
- Peats Ridge Festival—Glenworth Valley, Australia
- Pitchfork—Chicago, Illinois
- Power to the Peaceful—San Francisco, California
- Red Wing Roots—Virginia
- Rock the Green—Wisconsin
- Roskilde—Denmark
- Sweetlife—Columbia, Maryland
- SXSW—Austin, Texas
- Telluride Bluegrass Festival—Telluride, Colorado
- 10,000 Lakes Festival—Detroit Lakes, Minnesota
- Warmfest—Indianapolis, Indiana
- WOMAD festivals

GREEN HOME, greenhome.com

A resource for buying a variety of environmentally friendly products for your home.

GREEN MUSIC ALLIANCE, greenmusicalliance.org

An organization for music companies, artists, and fans to raise awareness about the environment.

GREENSEAL greenseal.org

A nonprofit organization that creates standards for sustainable products and services.

HEALTHY FOOD APPS I LOVE:
- Allergy Guard
- Food Tripping
- Fooducate
- Good Food Near You
- Harvest
- Is That Gluten Free?
- Locavore
- Nutrition Tips
- Seafood Watch
- Substitutions
- Superfoods
- True Food

IMAGINE THERE'S NO HUNGER, whyhunger.org/imagine

Yoko Ono Lennon and Hard Rock's approach to ending childhood hunger.

LITTLE KIDS ROCK, littlekidsrock.org

An organization dedicated to restoring and revitalizing music education in schools.

MEAT FREE MONDAY, meatfreemondays.org

Paul, Mary, and Stella McCartney's campaign to reduce the impact of meat production on our environment and health.

MIND GARDENS, mindgardens.org

Snoop Lion's nonprofit initiative to create sustainable, organic community gardens in Jamaica.

MOROCCAN ELIXIR ARGAN OIL, moroccanelixir.com

Argan oil blended with organic essential oils.

MY ECOLOGICAL FOOTPRINT, myfootprint.org

Determine your ecological footprint.

MULTIPURE WATER PURIFICATION SYSTEMS,

www.multipureco.com

The system I use and recommend to clients because it reduces the most toxins.

NARCOTICS ANONYMOUS (NA), na.org

A resource for those needing support with addiction.

NEW ORLEANS MUSICIAN CLINIC,

neworleansmusiciansclinic.org

A nonprofit group that provides health assistance to musicians and their families in New Orleans.

ONE, one.org

Bono's campaigning and advocacy organization whose mission is to end extreme poverty and preventable disease by 2030.

ORGANIC CONSUMERS ASSOCIATION, organicconsumers.org

Lists organic food companies and stores by state.

ROCK AND ROLL HALL OF FAME AND MUSEUM, rockhall.com

A museum dedicated to collecting and preserving music history.

SHFT, shft.com
Actor-rocker Adrian Grenier's lifestyle site for sustainable living through art, film, food, culture, and design.

SEAFOOD WATCH, seafoodwatch.org
Check for safety and sustainability of seafood.

SKIN DEEP, ewg.org/skindeep
A database that rates the safety of cosmetics and skin-care products and ingredients; a part of Environmental Working Group.

SLOW FOOD, www.slowfood.org
A nonprofit organization that brings awareness and events to the culture, diversity, and traditions around food and farming.

UN MUSIC AND ENVIRONMENT INITIATIVE (UNEP), unep.org
A nonprofit organization designed to "green" the music industry.

FAN CLUB

TWITTER
FACEBOOK   the Rockstar Remedy
NEWSLETTER   www.therockstarremedy.com
WEBSITE   www.therockstarremedy.com

MERCH

RxSTAR REMEDY SITE   www.therockstarremedy.com
THE HERBAN ALCHEMIST/ELIXIR STORE   www.theherbanalchemist.com
MOROCCAN ELIXIR   www. Moroccanelixir.com

READING RECOMMENDATIONS

D'Adamo, Peter, M.D., and Catherine Whitney. *Eat Right 4 Your Blood Type.* New York: Putnam Adult, 1997.

Golan, Ralph, M.D. *Optimal Wellness.* New York: Ballantine Books, 1995.

Hass, Elson M., M.D. *Staying Healthy with Nutrition.* Berkeley, CA: Celestial Arts, 1992.

Jones, David. *Textbook of Functional Medicine.* Gig Harbor, WA: Institute for Functional Medicine, 2006.

Petrini, Carlo. *Terra Madre.* White River Junction, VT: Chelsea Green, 2010.

Pitchford, Paul. *Healing with Whole Foods.* Berkeley, CA: North Atlantic Books, 1993.

Pizzorno, Joseph E., Jr., and Michael T. Murray. *Textbook of Natural Medicine.* Edinburgh and New York: Churchill Livingstone, 2012.

Pizzorno, Lara U., Joseph E. Pizzorno Jr., and Michael T. Murray. *Natural Medicine Instructions for Patients.* New York: Harcourt, 2002.

Rosenthal, Joshua. *Integrative Nutrition.* New York: Integrative Nutrition, 2007.

Singh, Dharma, M.D. *Food as Medicine.* New York: Atria Books, 2004.

Weintraub, Skye, N.D. *Allergies and Holistic Healing.* Pleasant Grove, UT: Woodland, 1997.

PLUS ANY TITLES BY:

Jeff Bland
Deepak Chopra
Thich Nhat Hanh
Mark Hyman
Dalai Lama
Carolyn Myss
Christianne Northrup
David Perlmutter
Eckhart Tolle

ENCORE!

would like to thank all of the people who have contributed to making *The Rockstar Remedy* possible. I've always dreamed of starting a revolution, one that would shift the paradigm of health to a platform that was accessible to those who never considered good health could be for them. Taking my message to this "new" audience was somewhat controversial in the conservative world of health books. The story of my journey in the music industry as a rock & roll doctor needed to be told and supported by the most unlikely health ambassadors . . . rock stars. The journey has been perilous, arduous, frustrating, synchronistic, enlightening, and joyful. And it would not be possible without the following contributors:

Let's give it up for . . .

THE AUDIENCE AND FANS Thanks to the readers, patients, and music fans who have dedicated themselves to making the changes necessary to live a life that balances great health with joy! Thank you for sharing your stories of healing with me. I am always honored to be your guide.

THE VIPS My deepest love goes to my family, who have always given unconditional love and have supported and encouraged my rebellious ideas and heart's desires: Ahmed Jeriouda, Patricia Francis, Ronald Francis, Gibran Francis, Najla Francis, Elsie Nicola, George Nicola, Shannon Francis, Daniel Francis, Nicole Francis, Rachel Francis, Paul Francis, Elizabeth Francis, Nathan Francis, Jean Francis, John Wilmot, Jamie Wilmot, Jackson Wilmot, Nicholas Brayer, Celeste Brayer, Seth Brayer, Robyn McGinty, Shelly Anthony, Jenny Anthony, Adele Anthony, Barbara Pete, Kathy Pete, Jeff Pete, Mike Pete, Diane Pete, Gina Nicola, and the entire extended Lebanese village of aunts, uncles, nieces, nephews, and cousins, cousins, and more cousins.

THE GROUPIES My friends have been my concert partners and celebrated my adventures in travel, music, medicine, and spirit: Robyn McGinty, Rita Jabbour, Rose Mucci, Sonya Kaleel, Laura Brown, Marta O'Connor, Tom Francescott, Dalia Carella, Monica Watters, Christine Strater, Phyllis Adams, Tina Awad, Rachel MacPherson, Jennifer Hickman, Dena Al-Adeeb, Gaye Nelson, Kris Romano, Lisa Reiger, Debbie Melnik, Eileen Kerr, Judy Mondry, Ellen Doran, Mary Lou Garmon, and Victoria Fernandez.

MY CREW The office assistants and essential "roadies" who keep my business thriving and growing, while keeping me healthy: Marta O'Conner, Robyn McGinty, Laura Brown, Julia Carlin, Natalie Rock, Diane Hutchinson, and Ahmed Jeriouda.

THE MANAGEMENT Thank you to the agents at Foundry Literary Agency who have taken this crazy idea and helped me make a book out of it: Peter McGuiggan, Brandi Bowles, and Yfat Reiss Gendell. I truly appreciate the opportunity you have given me. Thanks to the project managers who connected and contacted many of the cast in order to make a great proposal possible: Monika Tashman and Josh Zeiman. And thank you to the "godfather" of celebrity doctors, Richard Pine, who planted in my mind the seed to write a book.

THE PRODUCERS Thanks to Karen Rinaldi, Julie Will, Sydney Pierce, and their team at Harper Wave for believing in the message and taking the book to the audience who needs it most. Your enthusiasm and support are priceless!

THE PHOTOGRAPHERS Big thanks to the wildly eccentric and lovin' Mick Rock, and the very cool and down-to-earth Danny Clinch. Your photos tell us the stories of the idols we love and emulate your own souls. Also, thank you to my personal photographers, Mickey Pantano, Claudia Hehr, and Seher Sikander. You have captured my best!

THE JOURNALISTS Huge thanks to Lonn Friend for your amazing artist connections and interviews and for sharing your adventures of soul and spirit. Massive thanks to Juliet Panebianco, the "Human Magnet." You have done the most supreme interviews and generously shared and connected the most intriguing people in the universe. The work you have done has brought this book to life just like any event that is lucky enough to have you. Thank you both for sharing the synchronicity and serendipity . . . and the message.

THE SPECIAL GUEST APPEARANCES Big thanks to all the amazing artists and musicians who have generously contributed their stories, wisdom, and humor. You are truly the ambassadors of the Rockstar Remedy revolution. Your insights and stories make the message of health fresh and funky! Very big thanks to Michael Franti for writing the Opening Act . . . you are truly a living ambassador of peace, health, and the groove.

THE BAND   Biggest thanks goes to Stacy Baker Masand for your patience, generosity, organization, grace, and exquisite writing talents. You have taken my ethereal visions and dreams and made them into reality. I can never thank you enough!

IN MEMORY OF LOU REED, 1942–2013

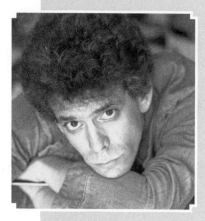

LOU REED
(MICK ROCK)

Lou Reed was and always will remain an iconic rock & roll legend known by many as the Father of Punk, Indie, and Alternative Rock. As a poet, writer, musician, and photographer, he inspired fans and musicians of all genres from his days with the Velvet Underground and continuing throughout his colorful career.

Lou lived the life of the extremes and excesses in the early years, but adventured on to have a productive and creative life into his early seventies despite a failing liver. Much of that he attributed to his tai chi practice.

We will always remember his rebellious spirit and the strength, power, and sincerity that he brought to rock & roll.

The King is gone but he's not forgotten . . .
—from *Rust Never Sleeps*, by Neil Young

INDEX

Entries in italics refer to illustrations.

oranges, 134
oregon grape root, 71
oregano, 71, 117
organic food, 11, 17, 18, 59, 103, 109–11, 113, 141, 143, 144
  labels and, 138–39
Orianthi, 226
Osbourne, Ozzy, xv, 10, 288
Ottolenghi, Yotam, 72
Our Lady Peace, 95, 107
outpatient treatment centers, 279
Overeaters Anonymous, 279
oxybenzone, 179
oxygen, 83

pain medication, 43
pancreas, 58
parabens, 179
parasympathetic mode, 170, 174
parsley, 71, 117
partially hydrogenated fats, 125
parties, 215–19
passionflower, 238, 254, 261, 262
pasteurization, 122, 123, 143
patchouli, 204
Peace Is Every Step (Thich), 84
peanut butter, 125
peanuts, 119
Pearl Jam, 19, 32, 130
pedometer, 156
PEGs, 180
pendulum swing, 25, 27, 35
pepper, 117
peppermint, 204, 243
personal care products, 38, 90, 293
personal inventory, 85–86
Persson, Nina Elisabet, 166, 273
pesticides, 39, 92, 109, 111, 128, 146
petroleum, 39, 92, 180
Pharmasan Labs, 285
phenylalanine, 116
phenylenediamine, 180
phosphatidyl serine, 261
phthalates, 180
phytochemicals, 18
phytonutrients, 107, 133
Pilates, 165, 166
Pilson, Jeff, 79, 249
Pink, 3, 75, 77
Pink Floyd, 112
Pirner, Dave, 270, 274
plantain, 271

plastic bottles, 92, 114, 115
plastics, 22, 39, 119
plastic surgery, 181–82
Plenty (Ottolenghi), 72
Pop, Iggy, 56, 69
Popoff, A. Jay, 151
pork, 113
positive attitude, 29, 137
potassium, 132, 247
poultry, 64, 105, 138, 144
prayer, 29, 86, 192, 207, 208
premenstrual syndrome (PMS), 124, 264–65
Preservation Hall Jazz Band, 17, *17*, 25, 150
preservatives, 108, 125
prickly ash, 71
Primal Defense, 228
probiotics, 66, 228, 234, 237, 243, 244, 256, 265, 269
protein, 42, 131, 132, 134, 206
protein bars, 136
proteolytic enzymes, 237, 240, 253, 266, 268
psoriasis, 43
psychoneuroimmunology, 11–12
psychotherapy, 86, 200–202, 251, 254
psyllium, 244

Qi, 160, 175
Q Prime, 201
Queensrÿche, 91, 227
Quiet Riot, xv, 10
quinoa, 133, 142

radiation, 90–91, 225–26
rashes, 43
Rebecca drink, 218
Red Bull, 130
red clover, 71, 244
Red Dye No.3, 137
red meat, 105, 113, 133, 143, 244
red raspberry leaf, 260
refined flours and sugars, 108, 140, 142, 145, 248–49
reflexology, 173
Reiki, 204–4, 249, 252, 267
relationships, 29–30, 38–39, 51, 83, 87–88, 195–98, 201–2
religion, 199–200, 207
R.E.M., 16, 19, 144, 205
REM sleep, 205
REO Speedwagon, 96, 187
repetitive stress injuries, 165

ABOUT THE AUTHORS

DR. GABRIELLE FRANCIS, *THE HERBAN ALCHEMIST*

DR. GABRIELLE FRANCIS has been practicing holistic medicine for more than thirty years. She is a naturopathic doctor, chiropractor, acupuncturist, and massage therapist.

In practice, Dr. Francis adheres to the philosophy and principles of naturopathic medicine, which include:

THE HEALING POWER OF NATURE

IDENTIFYING AND TREATING THE CAUSES

FIRST DO NO HARM

DOCTOR AS TEACHER

TREAT THE WHOLE PERSON

PREVENTION

Gabrielle received her formal medical training at National College of Chiropractic and at Bastyr University. She also has extensive training in alternative cancer therapies, environmental medicine, Functional Medicine, mind-body medicine, and bioidentical hormone therapies. Following her formal medical education, Dr. Francis traveled extensively to various parts of the world, studying medicine with indigenous healers in countries such as China, India, Thailand, Bali, Brazil, Morocco, Peru, Guatemala, Ecuador, Belize, Mexico, Egypt, and Mali. Gabrielle currently practices in New York City as the Herban Alchemist and operates Backstage Alternative, which provides natural medicine to rock & roll performing artists on tour.

STACY BAKER MASAND is a health, fitness, and lifestyle editor whose work has appeared in magazines such as *InStyle*, *Marie Claire*, *Self*, *Shape*, *Fitness*, *DuJour*, and *Women's Health*. She is the coauthor of the *New York Times* bestseller *Your Best Body Now* and is currently developing projects for both the small and big screen.